# The G-Jo Institute
# Manual of
# Medicinal Herbs

# The G-Jo Institute Manual of Medicinal Herbs

by Michael Blate

ROUTLEDGE & KEGAN PAUL
London, Melbourne and Henley

This book is presented as a catalog and primer of techniques and other information that have been in continuous use throughout the Oriental and Western world for many years. While these techniques and information utilize a natural system within the body, there are no claims made for their effectiveness, even when properly used. These techniques and information are not an alternative to proper medical care and treatment, nor are they intended to supersede or replace any standard, Western first-aid, emergency or medical techniques.

Illustrated by Michael Blate and Dover Publications

*First published in Great Britain in 1983*
*by Routledge & Kegan Paul plc*
*39 Store Street, London WC1E 7DD, England*
*464 St Kilda Road,*
*Melbourne, Victoria 3004, Australia*
*Broadway House, Newtown Road,*
*Henley-on-Thames, Oxon RG9 1EN, England*
*Printed in Great Britain by*
*Unwin Brothers Limited, The Gresham Press, Old Woking*
*Surrey GU22 9LH*

*British Library Cataloguing in Publication Data*

*Blate, Michael*
*The G-Jo Institute Manual of Medicinal Herbs*
*1. Herbs-therapeutic use*
*1. Title*
*615'. 321   RS 164*

*ISBN 0–7102–0029–3*

To the members of The G-Jo Institute, and to Dawna — teacher in her own, unique way and an awfully neat lady, as well.

"The body is a house given to you for rent; the owner is God.  Live there so long as He wills, thanking Him and paying Him the rent of faith and devotion."
Sri Sathya Sai Baba

# CONTENTS

## ACKNOWLEDGMENTS

The author wishes to thank and gratefully acknowledge the help and assistance of many members and friends of The G-Jo Institute. He is especially grateful to:

* Laurie Blate
* Al Fon
* Andrea Holly Gold
* Dick Knierim
* Sandy Pasquale
* Diane Ruby
* Barbara Sisson
* Jimmy Sullivan
* Sharon Tufaro
* Gail Watson
* Peggy Wells

# WHAT IS THE G-JO INSTITUTE?

The G-Jo Institute is a not-for-profit natural health research and educational organization. It was informally organized in 1976 and incorporated in 1982. Its purpose is the development and dissemination of drugless "self-health" information and techniques.

G-Jo is a simplified form of acupuncture without needles (or "acupressure"). However, the scope of The G-Jo Institute has expanded far beyond its original purpose of sharing only simple acupressure techniques.

It is our belief that it is the body-mind — and only the body-mind — which heals itself. For that reason, we now address ourselves to the entire spectrum of how to stimulate the innate self-healing mechanisms witihin the body-mind with simple, yet effective, self-applied techniques from around the world.

For further information or catalogs about our publications, recordings, workshops and such, send a business-sized, self-addressed stamped envelope to:

THE G-JO INSTITUTE
DIVISION H
POST OFFICE BOX 8060
HOLLYWOOD, FLA. 33024
U.S.A.

# A NOTE TO THE READERS

Herbal self-prescription is not recommended as a sole method of self-treatment. Nor should it be used in place of professional health care — a good doctor is a valued advisor and health counselor whose knowledge and services should be used when the need arises.

The information in this manual is based — as is nearly all herbal therapy — on both personal experience as well as folklore; its sources are believed to be reliable and sincere, but it should be used with common sense and consideration. If symptoms persist, see your doctor.

# INTRODUCTION

Nearly every habitable area of the earth has its own "broad-spectrum" medicinal herbs and plants. These typically have been used since before recorded history for healing and helping to prevent illness.

The study of herbs and their medicinal uses — called phytotherapy — has occupied many lives throughout the ages. Thus, no small book such as this could hope to present all the known information about any therapeutic plant, tree or fruit.

Instead, this work is presented as a primer and handy reference companion whose information should be used in conjunction with other "self-health" techniques (such as those presented in other G-Jo Institute-sponsored publications).

Good health is a complex process. Realizing this, the wise person uses any and all means available to restore and maintain this precious state of being. Being well is an ongoing adventure, but one that requires constant vigil. Throughout history, no self-healer has ever been considered "fully armed" without at least a cursory knowledge of the medicinal effects of a number of common herbal and nutritional substances.

My own self-health technique of choice is acupressure. Yet I have found that, on occasion, the knowledge and use of herbal remedies has proven itself beneficial. With this in mind, I welcome you to the following pages.

Michael Blate

## HOW TO USE THIS MANUAL

This manual may be used in three ways:

* As a reference to more than 70 commonly used medicinal herbs and plants;

* As a "self-prescriber" based on the <u>therapeutic action and qualities</u> ascribed to these herbs;

* As a "self-prescriber" based on the <u>symptoms or health disorders</u> you wish to treat.

To best use this manual, first scan Section I to acquaint yourself with the 73 herbal remedies and their many historical uses. Pay special attention to those symptoms which "fit" you and your family, noting those herbs which may be helpful. Then try to keep as many of those herbs on hand (it is not necessary to obtain <u>all</u> the herbs in this book — usually 20 or 30 are more than enough, since many of their qualities and actions overlap).

Then, when the need arises, turn to Sections II or III to find the most appropriate herb(s) for the "target" symptom(s) and use accordingly.

# ABOUT HERBAL REMEDIES

## HOW HERBS APPEAR TO WORK

The healing action of most herbs appears to be
somewhere between the profound-but-gross action of
<u>allopathy</u> (which includes most drugs and medicines
created by Western science and the pharmaceutical
industry) and the profound-but-subtle action of
<u>homeopathy</u> (which appears to work at the atomic level
of the human being).

Thus, most herbal remedies are safer — but
slower-acting — than either allopathic (yin-like, in
traditional Oriental philosophy) medicines or home-
opathic (yang-like) preparations.

Herbs appear to operate at a <u>cellular</u> level,
ultimately affecting the organ or gland most compatible
with that herb. (In the traditional Eastern philosophy
— which is the basis for this manual — each symptom
or ailment we suffer is considered to have an organ or
gland for its "home.")

And since a malfunctioning organ or gland may
manifest many different symptoms, one herb may relieve,
treat or heal a number of disorders.

Because allopathic drugs and medicines act quickly
and profoundly, there is an immediate sense of 'accom-
plishment"; the same is true for acupressure and other
"touch therapies" (See THE NATURAL HEALER'S
ACUPRESSURE HANDBOOK, available through the
G-Jo Institute — see address on page ix) — immediate,
if sometimes temporary, results. Herbs and other
"subtle" therapies take longer to show results; but
their results are broadly based and appear to work at
many "levels" at the same time.

## HERBS ARE SAFE YET EFFECTIVE

While herbs are medicinal, their action, generally speaking, is gentle and slow-acting. For this reason, herbs are usually safe for self-prescribing. Benefits should occur within three weeks to six months (for chronic problems) when using herbal therapy alone. One year is generally considered the safe, maximum limit for using the same herbal remedy or mixture.

But just as chemical medicines which are abused may have negative effects, so natural "medicines" (such as herbs) may also have the opposite of their intended effect if not properly used. This is especially true of herbs picked at the wrong time of the year or those improperly prepared (although you'd generally have to take them in unusually large quantities for any damage to occur).

So unless you're an expert in identifying and preparing medicinal plants, it is best to purchase them from a reputable source. And when buying herbs from a store or by mail, always check the Latin (botanical) name as well as the common name; often, a common name (such as "masterwort") may be applied to several different plants.

In the Orient, where the medicinal use of food and herbs has been practiced and recorded for thousands of years, it is said that nutritional therapy is only one important "leg" of a personal health-care program. The other parts needed to restore and maintain wellness are exercise, acupressure (or similar manipulative therapies), proper breathing, prayer and simple relaxation techniques (such as meditation).

You would be wise to follow the same path (many guides and learning aids are available through The G-Jo Institute).

# WHAT ARE "MEDICINAL HERBS?"

For the purposes of this manual, an herb is described as any plant, fruit or leaf, etc., which appears to manifest medicinal (healing) qualities While this could include nearly anything that grows (Tibetan healers — some of the most astute and advanced physicians in the world — ascribe medicinal qualities to virtually every substance on earth, including rocks, precious gems and such), this manual will address itself to only the more common and widely used medicinal plants.

There are numerous medicinal qualities that herbs may manifest (e.g., carminative, depurative, diuretic, etc.). In following sections, all the major medicinal qualities — as well as some of the most popular herbs which manifest them — are detailed for easy reference.

However, the medicinal qualities ascribed to these herbal substances are by no means their only qualities, nor are the bodily organs or systems they primarily affect the only parts of the body-and-mind ("body-mind") they reach. Herbal healing is both an art and an adventure — one that promises a life-long learning experience. And since each human being is unique, the pathway of discovering your own "ideal" herbal "formula" is always the blazing of a virgin trail.

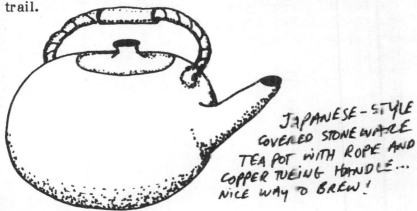

JAPANESE-STYLE COVERED STONE WARE TEA POT WITH ROPE AND COPPER TUBING HANDLE... NICE WAY TO BREW!

# HOW HERBS ARE USED

Most medicinal herbs have both internal and external uses. By far the most common use is internally, when the herb(s) are consumed as a "tea" or infusion.

Here, the blossoms and leaves are generally used, unless otherwise stated. Following the suggestions and recommendations below, one pint of boiling water is generally poured over one ounce or more of the plant substance, covered, and allowed to steep for a minimum of 30 minutes. Unless otherwise stated, herbal blossoms or leaves are never boiled.

A decoction is similar to an infusion. This preparation is made by boiling an herbal substance in water for a considerable period of time. Hard plant substances — barks, roots or seeds — are prepared in this manner, since they need longer exposure to heat to extract their medicinal qualities. Here, it is typical for one ounce of the herbal substance to be boiled (beginning with cold water) for a minimum of 30 minutes or longer in a pint or more of good water.

The "one ounce per pint" rule is a general one for medicinal use (when a strong infusion is ordinarily used). It might be less than this if you simply wish a pleasant-tasting, pleasantly scented beverage. As a mild, beverage-only infusion, herbs are generally safe to use beyond the one-year maximum limit. Of course, if you do notice any adverse reactions to herbal beverages, stop taking them.

## OTHER INTERNAL USES OF HERBS

Beside drinking them, another method of ingesting herbs is through inhalation — that is, being smoked in a pipe or cigarette. There are two times when herbal inhalation is recommended: To specifically affect the respiratory system; and as a "transitional bridge" for a person seeking to break tobacco addiction (see HOW TO STOP SMOKING WITH ACUGENCS, available from The G-Jo Institute).

Certain medicinal herbs may also be chewed and eaten — most notably garlic and ginger root, as well as similar, soft herbal bulbs or roots (e.g., ginseng, etc.). Here, the effects are most quickly manifested in the digestive (and perhaps the respiratory) system. These same herbs are often used in cooking, combining their seasoning with their medicinal qualities.

A fifth method of using herbs internally is to take an infusion as a "high" or retained enema. A strong herbal infusion is taken rectally and held for as long as possible, allowing the fluid to be absorbed through the walls of the colon, etc.

A less common and more complex method of extracting an herb's medicinal qualities is through a tincture. Pure or diluted drinking alcohol (e.g., brandy, vodka, gin, etc.) is used to "steep" the herb, using a mixture of 4 ounces of water to 12 ounces of the spirits and 1 ounce of the powdered herb.

This mixture is allowed to stand for 2 weeks or longer with the bottle being shaken regularly each night. The fluid is then strained and the sediment is discarded. A tincture is used in most cases when heat or water alone may not be sufficient to extract the medicinal qualities.

# THE EXTERNAL USE OF HERBS

Medicinal herbs may be used externally in a number of ways. One way is as a _fomentation_. This is a local application, usually of hot alternating with cool-to-cold large compresses moistened with a strong, herbal infusion. Their purpose is to relieve pain and increase circulation.

A cotton towel or similar thick cloth is folded to about 12 inches wide. Then a woolen blanket is placed on a table, while the cotton towel is saturated — up to 4 inches from either end — in the hot infusion, then laid onto the woolen blanket. This, in turn, is folded over the end so that one side has a double thickness.

The fomentation is then applied as hot as can be tolerated onto the affected skin area and left to cool. Run your hand under the fomentation on the skin as often as necessary to ease any heat discomfort. As the fomentation becomes more comfortable, lift it off and place a towel dipped in either cold water or cold herbal tea over the area for a minute or so. Then replace that with a hot fomentation again, as quickly as possible.

POULTICE —

EASY AND USEFUL FOR EXTERNAL APPLICATIONS...

HERBAL REMEDY ITSELF

PLASTIC OR SARAN-WRAP® FOR WET HERBS

CLOTH, HANDKERCHIEF, ETC., FOLDED ONCE OR TWICE

A poultice is a paste or 'package" of medicinal herbs which is laid onto an enlarged gland, abscess or other skin eruption. This is then covered with a layer of cloth (as well as, perhaps, plastic to prevent any leakage) and kept hot. The affected area should first be cleaned with hydrogen peroxide before applying the poultice.

Here, it is best to use powdered or granulated herbs, which may be mixed with corn meal or flaxseed meal — plus water — to make the paste. If fresh leaves are used, crush them first before applying.

Poultices are also used to: Relieve pain, congestion or irritation; to act as a disinfectant; to reduce inflammation; to bring a sore or boil to a head; to reduce swelling; to ease stress/tension; to stimulate skin healing; and to promote muscular relaxation. But it is generally best to avoid using a poultice on an area where pus has already formed.

Compresses are similar to — but smaller than — fomentations: these are hot, herbal tea-soaked cloths applied to an area of the skin. Cold compresses — or ice packs — may also be used alternately with the hot compresses.

An ointment is a condensed infusion, herbal extract or tincture mixed with a substance such as Vaseline® or other thick, "neutral" vehicle. It is rubbed and massaged — like a balm or liniment — into an affected skin area.

Each of these methods has its place for different kinds of symptoms. At least a cursory knowledge of these uses is helpful for anyone interested in herbal therapy.

# THE "CONSTITUTIONAL REMEDY"

The master herbologist (or herbalist) does not select one or several herbs for his patient lightly. This is because he realizes that each person suffers from a unique illness which is an expression of the sufferer's life-long constitutional weakness. He realizes that each disease can never be identical to a similar disease suffered by one's brother or neighbor, even though it might be called the same name and might have similar characteristics.

Furthermore, no part of a disorder or a disease can stand alone from any other aspect of the person who is suffering it. In other words, ideally a "cold" should not be treated without considering many other factors that preceded it.

To the master herbalist, there exists for each person a single, ultimate substance which, if taken properly, will cause a profound slowing and reversal of the sufferer's problem. This is called a "constitutional remedy."

But selecting the constitutional remedy is no easy task and requires an herbalist who is both knowledgeable and sensitive. Consequently, without many years of training and experience, it is unlikely any individual could accurately both diagnose — then self-prescribe for — his own condition.

# HOW TO SELECT THE RIGHT HERB FOR YOU

However, there <u>are</u> certain "rules of thumb" which may be helpful in selecting a good herbal remedy for your own symptoms. Whenever possible, choose that or those herbs that have the medicinal qualities you need and:

* Are grown locally;

* "Feel" intuitively right;

* Smell good (to you);

* Taste good or "right";

* Produce some noticeable benefits quickly;

* And which have been picked/prepared properly.

If in doubt about which herbs grow locally (within 50 miles of your home), contact your county agricultural agent. If he doesn't know, he may be able to direct you to someone who can help you. Then, from those, select the leaves or roots which taste best (or even <u>seem</u> best or somehow "right" for your problem — intuitive guidance can be a powerful force).

You will probably end up depending upon a small number of herbs. As mentioned, these should include primarily those which grow in your area, taste best, are easiest to obtain and which seem to produce the best results — rather than depending on all (or most) of the many herbs which are generally given for a specific symptom in the following pages.

If an herbal tea tastes <u>bad</u> and smells <u>bad</u> to you, don't use it; but if it smells good while tasting bad, it may be useful and helpful. And if it both tastes good and smells good, it may have far-reaching benefits beyond the "target" symptom(s).

# HOW TO PREPARE INFUSIONS AND DECOCTIONS

Always use stainless steel, glass, ceramic or clay utensils when preparing medicinal herbs. Never use aluminum, iron, lead or other toxic metals as these may not only change the herb or water's characteristics but may even be toxic, as well.

Begin by placing the dry herb(s) into a suitable pot or a proportional amount of that herb (about one large tsp. per cup) into a "tea ball" and place that in a cup. Now fill a kettle with cold, fresh water, then bring to a rapid boil. As soon as the water begins boiling, take it off the heat and pour it from as high as possible above the teapot (to restore the oxygen to the boiled water) over the leaves, blossoms and/or other "soft" parts of the herb. Now cover the teapot — no odor (which also tends to carry away some of the medicinal oils) should escape. Then let this infusion stand for 30 to 45 minutes to bring out the full medicinal qualities.

If making a decoction, place bark, twigs and/or roots in a stainless steel pot or pan covered with cold water. Cover the pot and bring to a rapid boil, then reduce heat and let simmer for at least half an hour. Drink either the infusion or decoction warm, but not boiling hot. Store any remaining liquid in the refrigerator to drink for a cool beverage instead of soft drinks or other fluids you might otherwise take during the day.

## WHAT HERBAL THERAPY SHOULD ACCOMPLISH

Herbs appear to accomplish their medicinal action by triggering a response in the "target" organs or glands that they reach. Ideally, an herbal therapy should accomplish at least three important functions:

* It should promote building, repairing and/or restoring of the malfunctioning organ or gland that it reaches;

* It should promote "elimination" of toxic residues of incomplete biochemical interactions (toxins) within those organs or glands;

* It should promote "balancing,' first of its target organ(s), then of the entire body-mind.

Be particularly observant for an adverse (allergic) reaction — this may include hives, rash or less noticeable effects, such as hyperactivity or irritability.

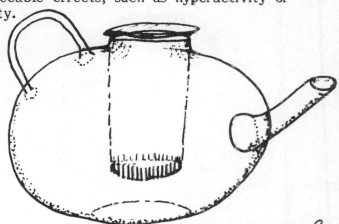

CLEAR GLASS TEAPOT MADE BY JENA OF WEST GERMANY... THE AUTHOR'S FAVORITE!

## ABOUT COMBINING HERBS

Herbs may be — and often are — combined for the purpose of broadening their medicinal qualities. However, usually not more than three, and never more than five herbs are combined (unless you are a skilled herbalist and are quite familiar with the effects you are creating). Remember: While each new herb that is added to the basic infusion may broaden its action, it also diminishes the medicinal action of the original herb(s).

In short, the more herbs and/or ingredients a tea or remedy has in it, the slower (but more broadly) it works. And the slower it works, the more suited it is for chronic problems — those which are of a long-standing nature and more greatly affect the entire person (as compared to an acute ailment).

Conversely, the fewer herbs and/or ingredients a tea or remedy has in it, the faster it works. And the faster it works the more suited it is to an acute problem or flare-up.

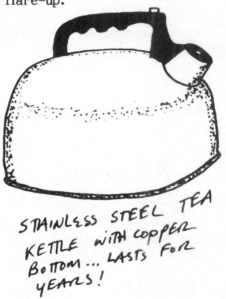

STAINLESS STEEL TEA KETTLE WITH COPPER BOTTOM... LASTS FOR YEARS!

# HERBAL "RULES OF THUMB"

Herbal therapy and especially self-prescribing is an imprecise art rather than a science. Few hard and fast rules exist. But if you don't notice positive results after three days of taking an herbal remedy for an acute problem, it's probably the wrong infusion or combination of herbs.

Please remember: Chronic problems take longer — sometimes several months or more — to manifest noticeable improvements when using herbal therapy, alone. The longer it took for a disease to manifest itself, the longer it takes for it to be "reversed" (healed).

Generally, four or five cups of the herbal infusion — or its equivalent, based on about one good-sized teaspoon of the loose herb per full teacup of water — are suggested to be consumed or used per day. Drink even more in the beginning of therapy, but gradually taper off after several months.

Historically, it is said when you find an herb or herbal combination that promptly improves a health disorder or disease, it is generally good for preventing a recurrence of that disorder when used less frequently. But if you don't feel any noticeable results within a few days after taking relatively heavy doses of an herbal remedy, then try another herb or combination.

Finally, there are several "don'ts" to remember: Don't use sugar to sweeten an herbal tea — if you must use any sweetening (and it's best if you avoid it), use only _raw_ honey. Also, don't take drugs and medicinal herbs together — they may cause a "cancelling" action to occur. Wait at least four hours between taking them (and preferably avoid one totally when using the other).

# HERBS CAN BE DANGEROUS

It is important to keep in mind that herbs <u>are</u> medicines. Even the most beneficial herbal remedies have the potential for abuse; and there are a number of dangerous herbs which should be generally avoided unless professionally prescribed. These include the following:

Jimson weed; daffodils; spurge; arnica; wormwood; scotch broom; devil's eye; buckeye; heliotrope (not the garden flower); mistletoe; periwinkle; wahoo bark; white snakeroot; yohimbe; spindle tree; mandrake; hellebore; squill; poison hemlock; tobacco (especially if used internally); tonka beans; aconite; white bryony; nux vomica; calabar beans; camphor (especially if used internally); ergot; ignatius beans; bittersweet; gelsemium; henbane; celandine; belladonna (deadly nightshade); castor beans (source of castor oil); foxglove (source of digitalis); mayflower; and any herb which produces an allergic reaction.

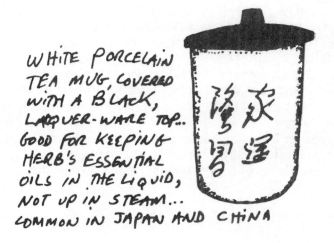

WHITE PORCELAIN TEA MUG, COVERED WITH A BLACK, LACQUER-WARE TOP... GOOD FOR KEEPING HERB'S ESSENTIAL OILS IN THE LIQUID, NOT UP IN STEAM... COMMON IN JAPAN AND CHINA

Even some of the herbs included in this manual — which are generally considered to be "safe" herbs — are potentially dangerous (that is, may be easily abused). Some of the popular, "potentially dangerous/use cautiously" herbs are the following:

Tansy (especially in large doses for pregnant women); rue; comfrey; valerian (this herb must never be boiled); pennyroyal (should be avoided by pregnant women); lobelia; golden seal; bloodroot; scullcap; lady's slipper; lily-of-the-valley; High John root; morning glory; calamus; black cohosh; blue cohosh and manzanita. Even ginseng — one of the "miracle" herbs from the Orient (as well as America) — may produce possibly dangerous symptoms if taken to excess (e.g., high blood pressure or hypertension, sleeplessness, skin eruptions, morning diarrhea, etc.).

The study of this, and other natural healing methods — such as those described in other Institute-sponsored publications — is one of the most exciting and rewarding learning experiences a person can have. Nearly always there are simple remedies for even complex problems if one will just obey and honor the natural laws which guide and rule our existence.

# SECTION I — BASIC HERBS TO KEEP ON HAND

* Alfalfa
* Aloe Vera
* Angelica
* Anise
* Bayberry
* Black Cohosh
* Blueberry
* Blue Cohosh
* Burdock
* Calamus
* Catnip
* Cayenne
* Chamomile
* Chaparral
* Chickweed
* Clover (red)
* Coltsfoot
* Comfrey
* Cubeb (berries)
* Damiana
* Dandelion
* Echinacea
* Elder
* Elecampane
* False Unicorn
* Fennel
* Fenugreek
* Garlic
* Ginseng
* Ginger
* Golden Seal
* Gotu Kola
* Hawthorn
* Hops
* Horehound
* Horsetail
* Hyssop
* Juniper
* Licorice
* Linden
* Lobelia
* Mandrake
* Marshmallow
* Masterwort
* Milkweed
* Mullein
* Myrrh
* Nettle
* Pennyroyal
* Peppermint
* Plantain
* Raspberry
* Rose, Rosehips
* Rosemary
* Sage
* St. Johnswort

* Sarsaparilla
* Sassafras
* Saw Palmetto
* Scullcap
* Self-Heal
* Slippery Elm
* Spearmint
* Tansy
* Uva Ursi
* Valerian
* Vervain
* Wintergreen
* Witch Hazel
* Wood Betony
* Yarrow
* Yellow Dock
* Sanicle

ALFALFA (Medicago sativa)

Also called: Lucerne; buffalo;

Part used: Leaves;

Primary medicinal qualities: Alkalizer; diuretic; stomachic; tonic; nutrient;

Affects: Teeth; digestive system; bowels; genitourinary system;

Often used internally for: Peptic ulcers; indigestion; bowel irregularities; addiction (to alcohol, drugs); weight imbalances; dropsy; lumbago; prostate disorders; genitourinary disorders;

Comments: A good all-purpose beverage (esp. when combined with mint) for general health.

ALOE VERA (Aloe socotrina)

Also called: Bombay aloes; Barbados aloes;

Part used: Gel from leaves;

Primary medicinal qualities: Cathartic; stomachic; aromatic; emmenagogue; drastic; vulnerary; emollient; antiseptic; tonic;

Affects: Digestive and reproductive systems; bowels;

Often used internally for: Constipation; indigestion; menstrual disorders; worms; bowel disorders;

Often used externally for: Sores; burns; insect bites; sunburn; skin disorders; hemorrhoids;

Comments: Powerful, broad-acting healer that is easy to grow at home.

ANGELICA (Angelica atropurpurea)

Also called: Masterwort; dead nettle; archangel;

Part used: Root; herb; seed;

Primary medicinal qualities: Aromatic; stimulant; carminative; diaphoretic; expectorant; diuretic; tonic; emmenagogue;

Affects: Respiratory system; digestive system; eyes; liver; spleen;

Often used internally for: Indigestion; heartburn; gas; colds and influenza; fevers;

Often used externally for: Eyesight/eye disorders (use as eye drops/wash); skin ulcers; ear drops;

Comments: A powerful healer with many uses.

ANISE (Pimpinella anisum)

Also called: Aniseed; sweet cumin;

Part used: Root; seeds;

Primary medicinal qualities: Stimulant; carminative; aromatic; diaphoretic; tonic; pectoral; relaxant; stomachic; flavorer;

Affects: Digestive system; respiratory system; chest; breasts;

Often used internally for: Gas/flatulence; colic; indigestion; nausea; rheumatism;

Comments: A pleasant-tasting (similar to licorice) herb that has many uses; especially helpful when mixed with fennel and catnip; seeds are often chewed after eating to aid digestion; increases breast milk.

BAYBERRY (Myrica cerifera)

Also called: Myrtle; wax myrtle; tallow shrub;
vegetable tallow; candleberry;

Part used: Bark (esp. bark of root); leaves;
flowers;

Primary medicinal qualities: Aromatic (leaves);
astringent; stimulant; tonic; diaphoretic; emetic
(large amounts); rubefacient; vulnerary

Affects: Glandular system; respiratory system;
digestive system;

Often used internally for: Diarrhea; chills (plus
cayenne); goiter; internal hemorrhage; poisoning
(narcotic); jaundice; leucorrhea; sore throat (gargle);

Often used externally for: Boils; styes; carbuncles;
sores; sore, bleeding gums;

Comments: A broad-acting herbal remecy.

BLACK COHOSH (Cimichifuga racemosa)

Also called: Rattleroot; squawroot; black snakeroot; bugwort; bugbane;

Part used: Root;

Primary medicinal qualities: Alterative; emmenagogue; diaphoretic; expectorant; nervine; astringent; antispasmodic; anodyne; diuretic; relaxant; sedative; tonic (for mucous membranes);

Affects: Respiratory system; circulatory system; female reproductive system; genitourinary system; liver;

Often used internally for: Rheumatism; pain; cough; whooping cough; spinal meningitis; asthma; poisonous snake, insect bites; hypertension; kidney disorders; liver disorders; childbirth (to ease).

Comments: A potentially dangerous herb which should not be consumed to excess.

BLUEBERRY (Vaccinium myrtillus)

Also called: Bilberry; whortle berry;

Part used: Fruit; leaves;

Primary medicinal qualities: Astringent (strong);

Affects: Spleen (fruit); endocrine system (fruit); lymphatic system;

Often used internally for: Diarrhea (leaves).

<u>BLUE COHOSH</u> (Caulophyllum thalictroides)

<u>Also called</u>: Blueberry; squaw root; blue ginseng; papoose root; yellow ginseng;

<u>Part used</u>: Root;

<u>Primary medicinal qualities</u>: Emmenagogue; diuretic; diaphoretic; antithelmintic; antispasmodic;

<u>Affects</u>: Genitourinary system; digestive system;

<u>Often used internally for</u>: Delayed/suppressed menstruation; easing childbirth; uterine disorders; rheumatism; vaginitis; hypertension; coughs; palpitations of heart; colic; hiccough; whooping cough; cramps; epilepsy;

<u>Comments</u>: Should be used with other similar-acting herbs, rather than alone. A potentially dangerous herb which should not be consumed to excess.

BURDOCK (Arctium lappa)

Also called: Clotburr; happy major; love leaves;
bardana; burr seed;

Part used: Root; seed; leaves;

Primary medicinal qualities: Diaphoretic; diuretic;
alterative; aperient; depurative; depilatory (root);
febrifuge; vulnerary; antispyhilitic;

Affects: Lymphatic system; kidneys; liver; blood
(root); skin; genitourinary;

Often used internally for: Gout; rheumatism; canker
sores; syphilis; sciatica; gonorrhea; indigestion; skin
diseases; falling hair;

Often used externally for: Burns; hemorrhoids;
swelling; wounds/injuries; sores/eruptions;

Comments: A broadly useful healer with many healthful
properties.

CALAMUS (Acorus calamus)

Also called: Sweet flag; sweet root; grass myrtle;

Part used: Root;

Primary medicinal qualities: Carminative; aromatic; tonic; vulnerary; febrifuge; stomachic; alkalizer;

Affects: Digestive system;

Often used internally for: Indigestion, gas, flatulence; improving appetite; fevers.

Comments: A potentially dangerous herb which should not be consumed to excess.

CATNIP (Nepeta cataria)

Also called: Catmint; catswort; nip;

Part used: Leaves; flowering top; whole plant;

Primary medicinal qualities: Anodyne antispasmodic; carminative; aromatic; diaphoretic; nervine; emmenagogue; refrigerant; stimulant; tonic; sedative;

Affects: Digestive system; nervous system; respiratory system;

Often used internally for: Indigestion; headaches; gas/flatulence; hyperacidity; pain; hysteria; coughs; colic; nervousness;

Often used externally for: Enemas;

Comments: A gentle, yet broad-acting balancer; nice taste and aroma.

CAYENNE (Capsicum annuum)

Also called: Red pepper; chili pepper;

Part used: Fruit;

Primary medicinal qualities: Stomachic; rubefacient; mucilaginous; pungent; nutrient; linament; styptic; alterative; sialagogue; stimulant; tonic; febrifuge; depurative; antispasmodic; sudorific; antiseptic; emetic; hepatic; diaphoretic;

Affects: Gastrointestinal system; respiratory system; circulatory system; liver; genitourinary system; spleen; pancreas;

Often used internally for: Digestive disorders; fevers; colds and influenza; rheumatism; constipation; shock; nasal congestion; coughs;

Often used externally for: Bleeding wounds; pleurisy; rheumatism; sore throat;

Comments: One of the most important broad-acting herbal remedies; as close to a "universal healer" as exists; even though pungent, may be eaten regularly and frequently without apparent harm, though should be consumed only in moderation by those on a spiritual pathway calling for low activity, meditation, etc; especially useful in the tropics and in hot climates.

## CHAMOMILE (Anthemis nobilis)

Also called: Ground apple; whig plant; low chamomile; Roman chamomile; camomile;

Part used: Flowers; upper part of plant;

Primary medicinal qualities: Anodyne; stimulant; stomachic; antispasmodic; carminative; tonic; vulnerary; sedative; relaxant; aromatic; bitter;

Affects: Genitourinary system; spleen; digestive system; nervous system; respiratory system;

Often used internally for: Bronchitis; colic; gallstones; earaches; nervousness; menstrual cramps; indigestion; nightmares; tinnitus; swollen glands; colds and influenza;

Often used externally for: Hair brightener (apply as rinse); injuries/wounds (poultice); eye wash;

Comments: A pleasant-tasting herb that makes a delicious beverage; medicinally, hard to abuse — gentle yet broad-acting.

CHAPARRAL (Larrea mexicana)

Also called: Creosote;

Part used: Entire plant;

Primary medicinal qualities: Antisyphilitic; antiseptic; laxative; alterative;

Affects: Blood; circulatory system; liver; genitourinary system; skin;

Often used internally for: Cancer; venereal diseases; arthritis/rheumatism; blood "cleansing"/purifying; LSD overdose; enemas;

Often used externally for: Sores/boils/ulcers (wash, rinse);

Comments: Often used during fast as a cleanser; because taste and smell are rather unpleasant, another method — perhaps less desirable — is the use of capsules/tablets.

CHICKWEED (Stellaria media)

Also called: Starweed; stitchwort; Adder's mouth; scarwort;

Part used: Whole plant; leaves (crushed, for poultice);

Primary medicinal qualities: Nutrient; alterative; vulnerary; demulcent; refrigerant; discutient; astringent; mucilaginous; pectoral; exanthematous; resolvent; laxative;

Affects: Respiratory system; digestive system; skin; circulatory system;

Often used internally for: Lung/bronchial disorders; hoarseness; colds and influenza; blood poisoning; constipation; inflammation;

Often used externally for: Tumors; problems with the testicles; burns/scalds; skin eruptions; sore eyes; hemorrhoids;

Comments: A garden "nuisance" with many beneficial qualities; often eaten like spinach; used as an herbal healer, internally and externally.

CLOVER (Red) (Trifolium pratense)

Also called: Cow grass; clever grass; marl grass;

Part used: Blossoms;

Primary medicinal qualities: Alterative;
antispasmodic; depurative; stimulant (mild);

Affects: Respiratory system; digestive system;
nervous system; skin;

Often used internally for: Nervousness; stomach
disorders; bronchitis; cough (esp. whooping cough);

Often used externally for: Wounds; sores; skin
ulcers.

COLTSFOOT (Tussilago farfara)

Also called: Bullsfoot; horsehoof; British tobacco; coughwort;

Part used: Leaves; flowers; root;

Primary medicinal qualities: Emollient; demulcent; expectorant; pectoral; diaphoretic; tonic; febrifuge (?);

Affects: Respiratory system; sinuses;

Often used internally for: Asthma; bronchitis; coughs; fevers; nasal congestion; hemorrhoids; sinusitis; safe tobacco replacer;

Often used externally for: Scrofulous tumors; sore throat (?);

Comments: Powerful but gentle effect on the respiratory system.

COMFREY (Symphytum officinale)

Also called: Knitbone; slippery root; knitback; healing herb; bruisewort;

Part used: Leaves; root;

Primary medicinal qualities: Astringent; antiseptic; demulcent; expectorant; mucilaginous; nutrient; styptic; vulnerary; pectoral; decongestant;

Affects: Respiratory system; liver; gallbladder; skeletal system; bones; skin; digestive system; bowels; genitourinary system;

Often used internally for: Bloody urine; anemia; any breathing disorder; cough; diarrhea; dysentery; hemorrhage; nasal congestion; laryngitis; menstrual disorders;

Often used externally for: Bruises; sprains; wounds; ulcers; boils, styes, carbuncles; swellings; abscesses; burns;

Comments: A powerful, broad-acting healer; it has numerous qualities but should be used in moderation (large prolonged doses have been associated with laboratory-produced cancer in mice).

CUBEB (BERRIES) (Piper cubeba)

Also called: Java pepper; cubers; tailed pepper;

Part used: Berries;

Primary medicinal qualities: Aromatic; stimulant
(mild); expectorant; stomachic; carminative; diuretic;
laxative; antisyphilitic; purgative;

Affects: Genitourinary system; digestive system;
respiratory system; bowels;

Often used internally for: Urinary disorders;
bronchitis; venereal diseases; gas/flatulence; colic;
cough; constipation.

DAMIANA (Turnera aphrodisiaca)

Also called: Mexican damiana;

Part used: Leaves;

Primary medicinal qualities: Aphrodisiac; aromatic; tonic; stimulant; laxative; nervine; bitter; stomachic; sedative;

Affects: Sexual/reproductive system; digestive system; bowels; nervous system;

Often used internally for: Increasing sexual drive; improving appetite; nervousness; fatigue, exhaustion, tiredness;

Comments: Often used with valerian, scullcap and/or saw palmetto berries.

DANDELION (Leontodon taraxicum; taraxicum officinalis)

Also called: Cankerwort; white endive; lion's tooth; puffball;

Part used: Root; leaves;

Primary medicinal qualities: Nutrient (leaves); aperient; depurative; diuretic; hepatic; stimulant; stomachic; tonic;

Affects: Digestive system; genitourinary system; glandular system; spleen; pancreas; liver; heart;

Often used internally for: Anemia; poor appetite; bowel inflammation; circulatory problems; edema; eczema; gas flatulence; diabetes; gallstones; digestive disorders; obesity; heart problems;

Comments: One of nature's own "miracle medicines."

ECHINACEA (Brauneria augustifolia)

Also called: Purple cove flower; Sampson root;

Part used: Root;

Primary medicinal qualities: Diaphoretic; alterative; depurative; antisyphilitic;

Affects: "Energy system"; genitourinary system;

Often used internally for: Venereal disease; any kind of blood poisoning (pus, gangrene; carbuncles, etc.);

Often used externally for: Sore throat (gargle); wounds;

Comments: Often combined with myrrh; also may be combined with elecampane to increase lung-healing benefits.

ELDER (Sambucus canadensis)

Also called: American elder; sweet elder; elderberry;

Part used: Bark; leaves; flowers; frui;

Primary medicinal qualities: Cathartic (bark and
berry juice in quantity); antisyphilitic emetic
(bark); alterative; discutient; diuretic; diaphoretic;
emollient; exanthematous; rubefacient; aperient;

Affects: Digestive system; bowels; genitourinary
system; liver;

Often used internally for: Constipation; urinary
disorders; epilepsy; diarrhea; colds; influenza; liver
disorders; venereal diseases;

Often used externally for: Burns and scalds; skin
problems; tumors; swellings.

ELECAMPANE (Inula helenium)

Also called: Scabwort; elfdock; wild sunflower;

Part used: Root;

Primary medicinal qualities: Alterative; aromatic; antiseptic; astringent; diaphoretic; diuretic; emmenagogue; expectorant; stimulant; stomachic; tonic;

Affects: Respiratory system; genitourinary system; reproductive system;

Often used internally for: Most lung/breathing disorders; delayed menstruation; kidney/bladder stones; fevers; urinary disorders;

Often used externally for: Skin (blemishes);

Comments: Often combined with echinacea.

FALSE UNICORN (Helonias dioica)

Also called: Helonias; drooping star wo⋅t;

Part used: Root;

Primary medicinal qualities: Emetic (large doses); sialagogue; stimulant; antithelmintic;

Affects: Digestive system; genitourinary system (?);

Often used internally for: Improving appetite; removing worms and internal parasites;

Often used externally for: Killing external parasites (e.g., lice, etc.).

FENNEL (Foeniculum officinale)

Also called: Wild fennel; sweet fennel; finkel; hinojo;

Part used: Seeds; leaves;

Primary medicinal qualities: Aromatic; carminative; diaphoretic; diuretic; pectoral; stimulant; stomachic; flavorer; bitter; refrigerant;

Affects: Digestive system; female reproductive system; liver; bowels; spleen;

Often used internally for: Gas/flatulence; colic; digestive disturbances (esp. in infants); gout; cramps; diabetes; fever; cough; obesity; rheumatism; snake/bug bites;

Often used externally for: Eye wash; painful swellings;

Comments: A gentle, broad-acting and pleasant-tasting healer; seeds are often chewed after eating a meal to aid and improve digestion.

FENUGREEK (Trigonella foenum graecum)

Also called: Bird's foot; foenugreek seeds;

Part used: Seeds;

Primary medicinal qualities: Farinaceous; tonic; carminative; mucilaginous; demulcent; febrifuge; arthritic; deobstruent; depurative;

Affects: Digestive system; bowels; circulatory system (?); kidneys;

Often used internally for: Fevers; stomach/bowel distress; sore throat; diabetes; blood poisoning; constipation (?);

Often used externally for: Sore throat; skin irritations;

Comments: Seeds are usually crushed — sometimes with Vaseline® and charcoal added for a poultice — before being used; often combined with aloe vera, anise, fennel, etc.

GARLIC (Allium sativum)

Also called: Common garlic;

Part used: Bulb;

Primary medicinal qualities: Antithelmintic;
antiseptic (do not place directly on skin);
aphrodisiac; carminative; digestive; diuretic;
expectorant; stimulant; stomachic; sudorific; tonic;

Affects: Virtually all systems of the body (and
particularly the spleen, pancreas, stomach and
kidneys);

Often used internally for: Coughs, colds and
influenza; poor appetite; food poisioning; infections;
sinusitis; respiratory problems of all sorts;
genitourinary disorders; male sexual stimulant; low or
high blood pressure; liver, gallbladder disorders;
gas/flatulence; menstrual and menopausal distress;
indigestion; dysentery and similar serious intestinal
disorders; cholera; improving strength; skin problems;
venereal diseases; constipation; depression; many heart
problems; preventive;

Often used externally for: Wounds (do not place
directly on open wounds, skin, etc.); hemorrhoids (use
like a suppository); external parasites (wear in a bag
around neck); skin problems (but do not place garlic
directly on skin — use a poultice);

Comments: Probably the "strongest," most widely
available, most popular of all herbal healers; however,
its use should be moderate for most people and
generally avoided by those of a "hot" or easily angered
nature or those on any spiritual pathway calling for
strict restraint, meditation, etc.

GINGER (Zingiber officinale)

Also called: Black ginger; African ginger;

Part used: Root;

Primary medicinal qualities: Aromatic; carminative;
condiment; diaphoretic (when taken hot); digestive;
emmenagogue; expectorant; pungent spice; sialagogue;
stimulant; stomachic; tonic;

Affects: Digestive system; repoductive system;
respiratory system;

Often used internally for: Delayed menstrual period;
cough; colds and influenza; indigestion; appetite
stimulation; gas/flatulence; backache; many lung
disorders; dysentery; diarrhea; bronchitis hangover;
improving circulation; nausea; headaches; sexual
stimulant and "balancer" preventive;

Comments: One of the most popular herbs in the
Orient, Thakkur calls it the "world remedy" — one of
the most precious herbs in nature. One of the small
handful of healing herbs whose use should be mastered.

GINSENG (Panax ginseng; panax quinquefolia)

Also called: Man's health; five-fingers; redberry;

Part used: Root;

Primary medicinal qualities: Preventative;
restorative; demulcent; diaphoretic; stimulant (mild);
stomachic; tonic; alterative; carminative; aphrodisiac;

Affects: Genitourinary system; circulatory system;
digestive system; nervous system; respiratory system;

Often used internally for: "Morning sickness"
(pregnant women); fevers; coughs; digestive disorders;
anemia; loss of appetite; constipation; depression;
headache; hiccoughs; insomnia; back pain; nausea;
rheumatism; low sexual vitality; low "energy";

Comments: One of the classic "miracle herbs", but
difficult to find truly medicinal-quality ginseng; the
best reputedly comes from Manchuria, then from Korea.
American ginseng is thought by many Chinese — the
originators of its use as a medicine — to be
relatively worthless, but American herbalists find
Western ginseng useful (albeit with fewer qualities
than ascribed to the Oriental varieties). A
potentially dangerous herb which should not be consumed
to excess.

GOLDEN SEAL or goldenseal (Hydrastis canadensis)

Also called: Tumeric root; yellowroot; orangeroot;

Part used: Root;

Primary medicinal qualities: Antiperiodic;
antiseptic; alterative; aperient; decongestant;
deobstruent; detergent; diuretic; laxative; vulunerary
opthalmic; stomachic; tonic;

Affects: Digestive system; liver; eyes; mucous
membranes; respiratory system; spleen; skin; bowels;

Often used internally for: Loss of appetite; nasal
congestion; colds and influenza; constipation; bowel
disorders; hemorrhoids; digestive disorders; prostate
problems; tonsillitis; "morning sickness" in pregnancy;

Often used externally for: Eczema eye problems;
mouth problems (use as mouthwash); inflammations;
sores;

Comments: A broad-acting and powerful healer which
should be used in moderation.

## GOTU KOLA (Hydrocotyle asiatica?)

**Also called**: Indian pennywort; march penny; ground ivy (?); fo-ti-tien; fo-ti;

**Part used**: Leaves;

**Primary medicinal qualities**: Anodyne; alterative; aperient; febrifuge; stimulant; narcotic (large doses); diuretic; antisyphilitic;

**Affects**: Bowels; nervous system;

**Often used internally for**: Rheumatism; fevers; increasing mental powers; bowel disorders;

**Often used externally for**: Venereal sores.

HAWTHORN (Crataegus oxycantha)

Also called: Haw; may; whitethorn;

Part used: Berries; seeds; root;

Primary medicinal qualities: Alterative; deobstruent;
laxative; stomachic; stimulant; nutrient; tonic (for
heart);

Affects: Digestive system; heart; circulatory system;

Often used internally for: Diarrhea; lumbago;
swelling of genitals; vomiting (root); nausea (root);
heart problems; digestive disorders;

Comments: When used as heart tonic, should be under
professional supervision.

HOPS (Humulus lupulus)

Part used: Flowers;

Primary medicinal qualities: Anodyne; antithelmintic;
diuretic; febrifuge; hypnotic; nervine; sedative;
stomachic; tonic; pectoral (?);

Affects: Liver; nervous system; digestive system;
discutient (?);

Often used internally for: Chest problems; throat
disorders; earache; toothache; digestive disorders;
nervous disorders; pain; neuralgia;

Often used externally for: Inflammation; boils;
tumors; skin irritations.

HOREHOUND (Murrumbium vulgare)

Also called: White horehound; marvel;

Part used: Flowers; leaves;

Primary medicinal qualities: Aromatic; antithelmintic
diaphoretic; diuretic; expectorant; hepatic; laxative
(large doses); pectoral; stimulant; tonic;

Affects: Respiratory system; reproductive system
(esp. females); spleen; liver;

Often used internally for: Throat disorders; coughs;
colds and influenza; expels afterbirth; promotes menses
which have suddenly stopped; breathing disorders;
expels worms.

**HORSETAIL** (Equisetum hyemale or hiemale)

**Also called:** Horsetail grass; shave grass; bottlebrush; paddock pipes;

**Part used:** Entire plant;

**Primary medicinal qualities:** Antithelmintic; astringent; depurative; diuretic; detergent; stomachic; decongestant; emmenagogue; hepatic; nervine; pectoral;

**Affects:** Genitourinary system; blood; nervous system;

**Often used internally for:** Many genitourinary dysfunctions; nasal congestion; hemorrhages; eye disorders (esp. opthalmia); copper poisoning (?);

**Often used externally for:** Bleeding wounds; swollen eyelids;

**Comments:** May become toxic under certain conditions or in excess.

HYSSOP (Hyssopus officinalis)

Also called: Holy herb.

Part used: Entire plant:

Primary medicinal qualties: Antiseptic; aromatic; aperient; antithelmintic; carminative; diaphoretic; expectorant; febrifuge; laxative; rubefacient; stimulant; sudorific; tonic;

Affects: Digestive system; genitourinary system; spleen; mucous membranes; throat; respiratory system;

Often used internally for: Coughs; colds; anemia; breathing disorders; epilepsy; blood pressure disorders (high/low); rheumatism;

Often used externally for: Healing cuts, wounds; insect bites and stings; sore throat (gargle); bruises (leaves); lice;

Comments: Often used with sage for respiratory problems (esp. as gargle for sore throat).

JUNIPER (Juniperus communis)

Also called: Juniper bush; juniper bark;

Part used: Berries: bark;

Primary medicinal qualities: Carminative; diuretic; stomachic;

Affects: Adrenals; genitourinary system; reproductive system (esp. female); respiratory system;

Often used internally for: Genitourinary disorders; colic; coughs; colds and influenza; digestive distress; gonorrhea; nervousness;

Often used externally for: Vaginal disorders (douche); insect bites (rinse);

Comments: Some authorities suggest avoiding juniper berries if you suffer from kidney disorders, while others suggest it as a remedy; in any event, use with caution and self-observation.

LICORICE (Glycyrrhiza giabra)

Also called: Licorice root; sweet wood;

Part used: Dried root; twigs; flowers;

Primary medicinal qualities: Demulcent; expectorant; laxative; febrifuge; stomachic; tonic; alterative; anodyne; flavorant;

Affects: Digestive system; respiratory system; liver, spleen;

Often used internally for: Digestive distress; cough; low energy; pain; fevers; thirst (has a cooling effect); throat/voice; increasing breast milk;

Often used externally for: Burns; boils; sores (most kinds, when mixed with honey and applied as salve);

Comments: One of the most widely prescribed/used medicinal herbs in the Far East; its sweet taste is often used to help other herbal compounds.

## LINDEN (Tilia platyphyllos)

Also called: Linden flowers; lime flowers; common lime; lime tree;

Part used: Flowers; leaves;

Primary medicinal qualities: Expectorant; diaphoretic; nervine; stimulant; stomachic;

Affects: Digestive system; respiratory system; nervous system; mucous membranes;

Often used internally for: Coughs; digestive disorders; menstrual distress; throat/voice;

Often used externally for: Boils; swellings; hoarseness (gargle);

Comments: Should not be confused with the citrus lime.

LOBELIA (Lobelia inflata)

Also called: Emetic weed; Indian tobacco; wild
tobacco; asthma weed; gagroot; eyebright;

Part used: Seeds; entire plant;

Primary medicinal qualities: Antispasmodic; diuretic;
emetic; expectorant; nervine; relaxant (large doses);
stimulant (small amount); diaphoretic; sedative;
pectoral; febrifuge;

Affects: Respiratory system; digestive system;

Often used internally for: Respiratory difficulties;
vomiting; heart palpitations;

Often used externally for: Pleurisy; pneumonia;
boils; swelling; bruises;

Comments: Should always be used with a stimulant,
such as cayenne; this controversial and powerful herb
borders on the category of "potentially dangerous" —
it should be used with caution, but has many
therapeutic qualities.

## MANDRAKE (Podophyllum peltatum)

**Also called:** May apple; hog apple; Indian apple; duck's foot;

**Part used:** Root;

**Primary medicinal qualities:** Alterative; antithelmintic; cathartic; deobstruent; diaphoretic; cholagogue; antibilious; resolvent; sialagogue; sedative; vermifuge; laxative;

**Affects:** Liver; bowels; reproductive system (esp. female);

**Often used internally for:** Coughs; angina; colic; liver/bowel regulator; liver disease (chronic); constipation;

**Often used externally for:** External parasites;

**Comments:** A poisonous herb in large quantities and an herb to be used with caution, moderation and for limited times, in any circumstances; professional guidance is suggested before using mandrake.

MARSHMALLOW (Althea officinalis)

Also called: Sweet weed; wymote; sweat weed (?);
althaea;

Part used: Root; leaves;

Primary medicinal qualities: Anodyne; demulcent;
diuretic; emollient; mucilaginous; opthalmic; pectoral;

Affects: Respiratory system; digestive system;
bowels; sexual organs; genitourinary system;

Often used internally for: Nasal congestion;
diarrhea; lung congestion; inflammation of digestive,
genitourinary tracts; respiratory disorders; pneumonia;
coughs; colds and influenza;

Often used externally for: Bruises; sprains; strains;
inflamed eyes (use as eyewash); vaginal irritation;

Comments: A gentle, broad-acting herb that is often
used with other "sweet" herbs or to sweeten up less
tasty infusions.

MASTERWORT (Heracleum lantanum)

Also called: Cow parsnip; youthwort; madnep;

Part used: Root; seeds;

Primary medicinal qualities: Carminative; diuretic; antispasmodic; stimulant; emmenagogue;

Affects: Digestive system; genitourinary system; respiratory system;

Often used internally for: Colds and influenza; fevers; delayed menstruation; kidney stones; epilepsy; asthma; palsy; apoplexy (stroke);

Often used externally for: Sores and ulcerations (rinse);

Comments: This herb should not be confused with any of the other so-called "masterworts": Angelica atropurpurea (angelica archangel) is covered elsewhere, while imperatoria ostruthium (imperial masterwort) has many similar qualities to heracleum lantanum.

MILKWEED (Asclepias syriaca)

Also called: Silkweed;

Part used: Root;

Primary medicinal qualities: Alterative; diuretic; emetic; purgative; tonic; laxative;

Affects: Bowels; genitourinary system; reproductive system (esp. female); liver; gallbladder; digestive system;

Often used internally for: Gallstones; genitourinary disorders; bowel disorders; asthma; stomach problems; poisoning (by mouth);

Often used externally for: Animal bites and stings.

MULLEIN (Verbascum thapsus)

Also called: Velvet plant; flannel leaf; bullock's
lungwort;

Part used: Leaves; flowers; root;

Primary medicinal qualities: Anodyne; antispasmodic;
astringent; demulcent; diuretic; emollient; pectoral;
vulnerary; sedative;

Affects: Respiratory system; bowels; skin;
genitourinary system;

Often used internally for: Coughs; colds and
influenza; respiratory disorders; diarrhea; nasal
congestion; rheumatism; bleeding in lungs; bowels; hay
fever; tooth disorders;

Often used externally for: Sore throat (gargle);
sores/wounds; warts (fresh, crushed flowers); toothache
(mouthwash); mumps; tonsillitis; glandular swellings.

MYRRH (Balsamodendron myrrh)

Also called: Gum myrrh;

Part used: Dried, Powdered Gum (Resin);

Primary medicinal qualities: Alterative; antiseptic; astringent; carminative; expectorant; emmenagogue; stimulant; stomachic; tonic; antispasmodic; vulnerary; pectoral;

Affects: Respiratory system; reproductive system (esp. female); mucous membranes; prostate; heart; digestive system;

Often used internally for: Rheumatism; gout; ulcers; hemorrhoids; cough; colds and influenza; respiratory disorders; delayed menstruation; leucorrhea;

Often used externally for: Gum disorders (e.g., pyorrhea — brush teeth with myrrh); sore/ulcerated throat (gargle); hemorrhoids;

Comments: An ancient yet invaluable healer with many uses.

NETTLE (Urtica dioica)

Also called: (Common) stinging nettle;

Part used: Entire plant;

Primary medicinal qualities: Anodyne; astringent; diuretic; febrifuge; pectoral; rubefacient; styptic; tonic; antithelmintic;

Affects: Respiratory system; genitourinary system (esp. kidneys); bowels; reproductive system (esp. female);

Often used internally for: Rheumatism; asthma (and most other respiratory ailments); hemorrhage (esp. within the genitourinary/reproductive systems); colds and influenza; diarrhea; fevers; hemorrhoids; neuralgia; obesity; poisonous bites/stings; baldness (alopecia); kidney stones; backache;

Often used externally for: Hemorrhage/bleeding (poultice of boiled leaves); dandruff; pain (poultice).

PENNYROYAL (Hedeoma pulegioides)

Also called: Squawmint; tickweed; hedeoma;

Part used: Entire plant;

Primary medicinal qualities: Aromatic; carminative; diaphoretic; emmenagogue; sedative; stimulant; sudorific; expectorant; febrifuge;

Affects: Digestive system; respiratory system; reproductive system (female); skin;

Often used internally for: Digestive disorders; nausea; vomiting; gout; headaches; toothache; delayed menstruation; colic; fevers; flatulence; poisonous bites/stings; skin disorders;

Often used externally for: Repels fleas and similar insects (esp. oil); mouth sores (rinse); bruises; skin disorders;

Comments: A potentially dangerous herb which should not be consumed to excess. Should be avoided by pregnant women.

PEPPERMINT (Mentha Piperita)

Also called: Brandy mint; lammint; balm mint;

Part used: Leaves; flowering tops;

Primary medicinal qualities: Aromatic; astringent;
antispasmodic; antiseptic; carminative; sudorific;
stimulant; stomachic; alterative (?);

Affects: Gastrointestinal system; bowels;
respiratory system; heart; circulatory system;

Often used internally for: Gas/flatulence; digestive
disorders; nausea; colic; diarrhea; fever; palpitations; colds and influenza; disorders of the nose,
throat; dizziness;

Often used externally for: Rheumatism; neuralgia;

Comments: An important therapy for the digestive
tract and one of the most basic of all herbs.

PLANTAIN (Plantago major or lanceolate)

Also called: Waybread; ribwort; ribworth; soldier's herb;

Part used: Leaves; root; fruit/seeds;

Primary medicinal qualities: Alterative; antisyphilitic; antiseptic; astringent diuretic; deobstruent; refrigerant; styptic; vulnerary; mucilaginous (seeds); sedative (seeds);

Affects: Genitourinary system; skin reproductive organs; liver;

Often used internally for: Rheumatism; wasting diseases; difficult labor; promoting fertility (esp. for strengthening male semen); kidney/bladder stones; bed-wetting; diarrhea; genitourinary disorders;

Often used externally for: Hemorrhoids; cuts; scratches; burns; sore eyes (rinse); eczema;

Comments: This common "pest" is one of the most broad-acting, widely used and easily obtained healing herbs.

RASPBERRY (Rubus stingosus or strigosus)

Also called: Red raspberry;

Part used: Leaves; fruit; (bark of) root;

Primary medicinal qualitites: Astringent; alkalizer
(fruit); alterative; antiemetic; laxative (fruit);
purgative; stimulant; stomachic; tonic; nutrient
(fruit);

Affects: Digestive system; genitourinary system;
bowels; gallbladder; liver; reproductive organs (esp.
female);

Often used internally for: Diarrhea (esp. in
infants); nausea; vomiting; difficult/painful
labor; slowing menstrual flow; sore throat;

Often used externally for: Bleeding cuts, wounds
(rinse).

ROSE, ROSEHIPS (Rosaceae)

Also called: Rosehips;

Part used: Fruit;

Primary medicinal qualities: Nutrient; astringent; pectoral; refrigerant; sedative; opthalmic (rose water);

Affects: Digestive system; respiratory system bowels;

Often used internally for: Coughs; colds and influenza; diarrhea; kidney stones (?);

Comments: An excellent natural source of vitamins C and P (bioflavinoids).

ROSEMARY (Rosmarinus officinalis)

Also called: Garden rosemary;

Part used: Leaves; flowers;

Primary medicinal qualities: Antispasmodic; aromatic;
astringent; carminative; diaphoretic; cephalic;
emmenagogue; nervine; stimulant; stomachic; tonic;
opthalmic;

Affects: Genitourinary system; digestive system;
reproductive system (esp. female); nervous system;
circulatory system;

Often used internally for: Colds and influenza;
cough; nervousness; headaches; baldness (alopecia);
depression; digestive disorders; circulatory problems;
anemia; menstrual disorders;

Often used externally for: Tooth and mouth disorders
(mouthwash); bad breath (mouthwash and gargle); sore
throat; eye problems (eyewash); shampoo;

Comments: Also a useful cooking herb.

SAGE (Salvia officinalis)

Also called: Garden sage; golden sage;

Part used: Leaves;

Primary medicinal qualities: Antiseptic; aromatic;
antispasmodic; carminative; diaphoretic (when taken
hot); diuretic (when taken cool); expectorant; nervine;
stimulant; sudorific; tonic; rubefacient; vermifuge;
antithelmintic; astringent; antiemetic; bitter;

Affects: Digestive system; genitourinary system;
reproductive system; liver; gallbladder; bowels;

Often used internally for: Kidney/genitourinary
disorders; liver/gallbladder disorders; gas/flatulence;
tiredness; nervousness; sexual balancing (esp. to
reduce excess sexual desire); fevers (esp. if high,
delerious — enemas); digestive disorders; beverage
(either hot or cool — see comments);

Often used externally for: Wounds/injuries
(superficial — wash with tea); sore throat/mouth sores
(gargle); baldness (alopecia — hair rinse); dandruff
(rinse);

Comments: An important basic herb and cooking spice;
IT SHOULD NOT BE BOILED (only steeped in hot water).

## ST. JOHNSWORT (Hypericum perforatum)

**Also called:** Johnswort;

**Part used:** Flowering tops; seeds;

**Primary Medicinal Qualities:** Aromatic; astringent; diuretic; nervine; resolvent; sedative; vulnerary; alterative;

**Affects:** Reproductive system (esp. female); blood; circulatory system; genitourinary system; bowels; nervous system;

**Often used internally for:** Blood "purifying"; tumors; boils/styes/carbuncles; uterine disorders; pus in urine; nervousness; bed-wetting; diarrhea; snakebite;

**Often used externally for:** Bruises (esp. as an ointment); caked breasts (ointment); scratches; bites and stings; skin irritations.

SANICLE (Sanicula marilandica)

Also called: Wood sanicle; black saricle; black snake root;

Part used: Root; leaves;

Primary medicinal qualitites: Alterative; astringent; depurative; discutient; expectorant; vulnerary; antisyphilitic; styptic;

Affects: Respiratory system; reproductive system (esp. female); genitourinary system; digestive system; skin; bowels;

Often used internally for: Venereal diseases; wounds (internal/external); ulcers/bleeding openings; tumors; tuberculosis;

Often used externally for: Sore throat/mouth sores (gargle); wounds; tumors;

Comments: A powerful internal and external healer — nearly a "cure-all" (according to Kloss).

SARSAPARILLA (Smilax officinalis, also aralia racemosa)

Also called: Jamaica sarsaparilla; spikenard; spignet;

Part used: Root; stalk; plant;

Primary medicinal qualities: Alterative; antisyphilitic; demulcent; diuretic; stimulant; carminative; sudorific (as hot tea); opthalmic; tonic;

Affects: Glandular/hormonal system; digestive system; respiratory system; skin; blood; circulatory system; genitourinary system; eyes; liver;

Often used internally for: Nasal congestion; colds and influenza; fevers; rheumatism/arthritis/gout; difficult/painful childbirth; skin eruptions; internal inflammations; ringworm; gas/flatulence; poison antidote (yin or yang poisons?): venereal diseases; eczema; heart disorders; improving eyes/eyesight (?);

Often used externally for: Tired sore eyes (eyewash); venereal diseases in newborns or infants (rinse).

SASSAFRAS (Sassafras officinale or laurus sassafras)

Also called: Cinnamon wood; saxafrax;

Part used: Bark or root;

Primary medicinal qualities: Alterative; aromatic;
antiseptic; diaphoretic; diuretic; flavorant;
stimulant; anodyne; febrifuge; stomachic; carminative;

Affects: Blood; circulatory system; digestive system;
bowels; genitourinary system; respiratory system;

Often used internally for: Arthritis/rheumatism;
pain; gas/flatulence; digestive disorders; colic; sore
throat; toothache (oil); skin diseases/eruptions;

Often used externally for: Skin diseases/eruptions;
ulcerated varicose veins;

Comments: Science has linked excessive use with
certain types of cancer in mice; may be difficult to
find in stores — but might be sold as room deodorizer.
In any event, this herb should be used in moderation
only.

## SAW PALMETTO (Serenoa serrulata)

**Also called**: Dwarf palm; dwarf palmetto;

**Part used**: Berries (fresh or dried);

**Primary medicinal qualities**: Antiseptic; sedative;

**Affects**: Respiratory system; genitourinary system;

**Often used internally for**: Respiratory ailments; genitourinary disorders; cough; colds and influenza; heart problems; sore throat; reproductive ailments; diabetes.

SCULLCAP (scutellaria lateriflora)

Also called: Blue pimpernel; mad weed; blue scullcap; hoodwort;

Part used: Entire plant;

Primary medicinal qualities: Antispasmodic; diuretic; nervine; tonic;

Affects: Nervous system;

Often used internally for: Arthritis/rheumatism; headaches (nervous); neuralgia; insomnia; nervousness; quinine-substitute; epilepsy; animal, insect and/or snakebite.

Comments: A potentially dangerous herb which should not be consumed to excess.

SELF-HEAL (Prunella vulgaris)

Also called: Wound wort; prunella (?); allheal;
healall; sicklewort;

Part used: Entire plant; stalks; leaves;

Primary medicinal qualities: Astringent; bitter;
antispasmodic; diuretic; stypic; tonic; vermifuge;
vulnerary; refrigerant (?); alterative; febrifuge;
pungent;
Affects: Respiratory system; liver; circulatory
system; gallbladder; skin;

Often used internally for: Fevers; wounds of all
sorts; arthritis/rheumatism; internal bleeding;
convulsions; obstructed liver; external bleeding;
bleeding ulcers (?); worms/parasites;

Often used externally for: Sore throat/mouth ulcers
(gargle); leucorrhea (douche); bleeding wounds, sores
(rinse/poultice).

SLIPPERY ELM (Ulmus fulva)

Also called: Red elm; moose elm; sweet elm; rock elm; Indian elm;

Part used: Inner bark;

Primary medicinal qualities: Demulcent; diuretic; expectorant; emollient; mucilaginous; nutrient;

Affects: Respiratory system; bowels; genitourinary system; digestive system; liver;

Often used internally for: Coughs; colds and influenza; respiratory ailments; digestive disorders; ulcers; inflammation of mucous membranes; sore throat; diarrhea;

Often used externally for: Sore throat (gargle); tumors/growths (esp. of womb); leucorrhea (douche); caked breasts; abscesses; skin irritations.

SPEARMINT (Mentha spicata or mentha viridis)

Also called: Garden mint; lamb mint; green mint;

Part used: Leaves; stems/stalks;

Primary medicinal qualities: Antispasmodic; aromatic;
carminative; diaphoretic; diuretic; stimulant;
stomachic;

Affects: Digestive system; bowels; genitourinary
system;

Often used internally for: Gas/flatulence; diarrhea;
digestive disturbances; hiccups; nausea; spasms;
urinary bladder stones; genitourinary inflammations;
vomiting (esp. in pregnancy);

Often used externally for: Hemorrhoids/piles;

Comments: A useful healer that should never be
boiled.

TANSY (Tanacetum vulgare)

Also called: Bitter buttons; yellow buttons; hindheel; mugwort (?);

Part used: Entire plant; seeds;

Primary medicinal qualities: Aromatic; bitter; diaphoretic; emmenagogue; stimulant; tonic; carminative (?); antithelmintic (?); vermifuge (seed);

Affects: Digestive system; bowels; reproductive system (esp. female); circulatory system; heart; genitourinary system; skin;

Often used internally for: Colds and influenza; delayed menstruation; fever; hypertension (high blood pressure); digestive disorders; kidney problems; heart palpitations; weak veins; worms;

Often used externally (esp. as fomentations or wet compresses) for: Tumors; swellings; inflammations; burns; sunburns; bruises; inflamed eyes; toothaches; freckles; pain (esp. low back pain);

Comments: A powerful healer but potentially dangerous; should be avoided especially by pregnant women.

UVA URSI (Arctostaphylos uva ursi)

Also called: Bearberry; bear grape; wild cranberry; arberry;

Part used: Leaves;

Primary medicinal qualities: Astringent; diuretic; tonic;

Affects: Genitourinary system; spleen; reproductive system; pancreas; liver;

Often used internally for: Kidney disorders; genitourinary ailments; diabetes; excessive menstruation; hemorrhoids; venereal diseases;

Often used externally for: Vaginitis, etc. (douche).

<u>VALERIAN</u> (Valeriana officinalis)

<u>Also called</u>: Vandal root; setwell;

<u>Part used</u>: Root;

<u>Primary medicinal qualities</u>: Anodyne; aromatic; antispasmodic; bitter; carminative; nervine; rubefacient; sedative; stimulant; tonic;

<u>Affects</u>: Digestive system; <u>nervous system</u>; <u>brain</u>; genitourinary system; bowels; liver;

<u>Often used internally for</u>: Memory loss/dysfunction; convulsions (esp. in infants); neuralgia; epilepsy; insomnia; heart palpitations; ulcers (stomach); pain; nervousness; genitourinary disorders (esp. stones);

<u>Often used externally for</u>: Wounds; sores; pimples;

<u>Comments</u>: A powerful — and potentially dangerous — healer whose primary qualities are of a calming, soothing nature; <u>DO NOT BOIL VALERIAN ROOT</u>!

VERVAIN (Verbena hastata; verbena officinalis)

Also called: American vervain; Indian hyssop; wild
hyssop;

Part used: Entire plant;

Primary medicinal qualities: Antithelmintic;
antispasmodic; astringent; decongestant; deobstruent;
depurative; diaphoretic; emmenagogue; expectorant;
emetic; nervine; sudorific; tonic; vermifuge;
vulnerary; febrifuge;

Affects: Blood; circulatory system; skin; respiratory
system; nervous system; reproductive system (esp.
female); genitourinary system; digestive system;

Often used internally for: Respiratory problems;
delayed menses; fevers; colds and influenza; epilepsy;
nervousness; skin disorders; insomnia; digestive
disturbances; worms/internal parasites;

Often used externally for: Sores; wounds;

Comments: A most powerful healer with numerous uses.

WINTERGREEN (Gaultheria procumbens)

Also called: Periwinkle; spiceberry; deerberry;
teaberries;

Part used: Entire plant;

Primary medicinal qualities: Antiseptic; astringent;
diuretic; emetic; emmenagogue; stimulant; carminative
(?); styptic;

Affects: Heart; circulatory system; digestive system;
genitourinary system; bowels; skin; sexual organs;

Often used internally for: Arthritis/rheumatism;
colic; gas/flatulence; diabetes; skin disorders;
venereal diseases (esp. gonorrhea); digestive
disturbances; bowel obstructions; back pains;

Often used externally for: For liniments of all
sorts; bleeding wounds; animal/insect bites;

Comments: Wintergreen should be used in small doses.

WITCH HAZEL (Hamamelis virginica)

Also called: Hazelnut; winter bloom; pistachio; tobacco wood;

Part used: Bark; leaves;

Primary medicinal qualities: Astringent; febrifuge; sedative; tonic; styptic;

Affects: Circulatory system; bowels; genitourinary system; reproductive system (esp. female); liver; spleen;

Often used internally for: Excessive menstruation; diarrhea; internal bleeding/hemorrhage; gonorrhea;

Often used externally for: Bruises; diarrhea (enema); painful tumors; gonorrhea; nosebleed (tea snuffed up nose); inflammations; piles/hemorrhoids; sores; sore throat (gargle).

WOOD BETONY (Betonica officinalis)

Also called: Lousewort; betony;

Part used: Leaves;

Primary medicinal qualities: Aperient; nervine;
stomachic; tonic; deobstruent; carmirative;

Affects: Bowels; liver; spleen; digestive system;

Often used internally for: Neuralgia; hangover (and
other effects of alcohol); stomach problems; digestive
disorders; obstructions of liver, spleen; colds and
influenza; worms/internal parasites; convulsions;
arthritis/gout; poisonous snakebite; headache;
biliousness; jaundice; facial/head pains; quinine
substitute/alternative; heartburn; colic;
delerium/insanity.

## YARROW (Achillea millefolium)

Also called: Milfoil; ladies' mantle; thousand leaf;

Part used: Entire plant;

Primary medicinal qualities: Alterative; astringent; diaphoretic; diuretic; stimulant; tonic vulnerary; aromatic (?); sudorific (?); febrifuge;

Affects: Circulatory system; genitourinary system; reproductive system (esp. female); spleen; bowels;

Used internally for: Colds and influenza; diarrhea; diabetes; fevers; internal bleeding/hemorrhage (esp. lungs, bowels); scanty/suppressed urine; measles; piles/hemorrhoids; small pox; chicken pox; digestive disorders; mucous membranes; gas/flatulence; quinine alternative; Bright's disease;

Often used externally for: Burns (rinse); piles/hemorrhoids; vaginal/menstrual disorders (douche); mouthwash; ulcers; wounds.

YELLOW DOCK (Rumex crispus)

Also called: Sour dock; curled dock; narrow dock.

Part used: Root;

Primary medicinal qualities: Alterative; astringent;
detergent; depurative; discutient; antiseptic;
vermifuge; demulcent; antisyphilitic;

Affects: Skin; circulatory system;

Often used internally for: Glandular tumors;
swellings; "impure" blood; itching; sores; cancer;
eruptive diseases;

Often used externally for: Tumors; swellings.

# SECTION II — HERBAL MEDICINAL QUALITIES

ALKALIZER: Neutralizes excess stomach acid; creates an alkaline condition within the body (generally considered healthful);

Herbs exhibiting this quality: Alfalfa; calamus; raspberry (fruit).

\* \* \*

ALTERATIVE: Purifies the blood; improves and gradually changes conditions for the better;

Herbs exhibiting this quality: Burdock; cayenne; chaparral; chickweed; clover; black cohosh; echinacea; elder; elecampane; ginseng; golden seal; gotu kola; hawthorn; licorice; mandrake; milkweed; myrrh; peppermint (?); plantain; raspberry; St. Johnswort; sanicle; sarsaparilla sassafras; self-heal; yarrow; yellow dock.

\* \* \*

ANODYNE: Relieves pain;

Herbs exhibiting this quality: Catnip; chamomile; black cohosh; gotu kola; hops; licorice; marshmallow; mullein; nettle; sassafras; valerian.

* * *

ANTIBILIOUS: Controls/eases the flow of excess bile;

Herbs exhibiting this quality: Mandrake.

* * *

ANTIEMETIC: Stops vomiting; soothes nausea;

Herbs exhibiting this quality: Raspberry; sage.

* * *

ANTIPERIODIC: Prevents return of periodic paroxysms; intermittent fevers, etc;

Herbs exhibiting this quality: Golden seal.

* * *

ANTISEPTIC: Counters putrefaction;

Herbs exhibiting this quality: Aloe vera; cayenne; chaparral; comfrey; elecampane; garlic; golden seal; hyssop; lobelia; myrrh; peppermint; plantain; sage; sassafras; saw palmetto berries; wintergreen; yellow dock.

* * *

ANTISPASMODIC: Stops/relieves/prevents spasms;

Herbs exhibiting this quality: Catnip; cayenne; chamomile; clover; black cohosh; blue cohosh; masterwort; mullein; myrrh; peppermint; rosemary; sage; scullcap; self-heal; spearmint; valerian; vervain.

* * *

ANTISYPHILITIC: Affects/relieves/helps to heal venereal
diseases;

Herbs exhibiting this quality: Burdock; chaparral
cubeb berries; echinacea; elder; gotu kola; (esp.
applied on venereal sores); plantain; sanicle;
sarsaparilla; yellow dock.

* * *

ANTITHELMINTIC; ANTHELMINTIC: Expels worms;

Herbs exhibiting this quality: Blue cohosh; false
unicorn; garlic; hops; horehound; horsetail; hyssop;
mandrake; nettle; sage; tansy (?); vervain.

* * *

APERIENT: Mildly laxative (a liver tonic); cleans
without harsh purgings;

Herbs exhibiting this quality: Burdock; dandelion;
elder; golden seal; gotu kola; hyssop. wood betony.

* * *

APHRODISIAC: Stimulates sexual desire;

Herbs exhibiting this quality: Damiana; garlic (esp.
males); ginger; ginseng.

* * *

AROMATIC: Mildly stimulating and has a pleasant smell;

Herbs exhibiting this quality: Aloe vera; angelica; anise; bayberry (leaves); calamus; catnip; chamomile; cubeb berries; damiana; elecampane; fennel; ginger; horehound; hyssop; pennyroyal; peppermint; rosemary; sage; St. Johnswort; sassafras; spearmint; tansy; valerian; yarrow (?).

*   *   *

ASTRINGENT: Causes contraction; stops discharges; draws tissue together;

Herbs exhibiting this quality: Bayberry; blueberry; chaparral; chickweed; black cohosh; comfrey; elecampane; horsetail; mullein; myrrh; nettle; peppermint; plantain; raspberry; rose/rose hips; rosemary; sage; St. Johnswort; sanicle; self-heal; uva ursi; vervain; wintergreen; witch hazel; yarrow; yellow dock.

*   *   *

BITTER: Improves appetite; more a quality — stimulating to the appetite — than a specific taste;

Herbs exhibiting this quality: Chamomile; damiana; fennel; sage; self-heal; tansy; valerian.

*   *   *

CARMINATIVE: Expels gas from entire digestive/
elimination tract; works primarily/secondarily on the
liver;

Herbs exhibiting this quality: Angelica; anise;
calamus; catnip; chamomile; cubeb berries; fennel;
fenugreek; garlic; ginger; ginseng; hyssop; juniper
berries; masterwort, mint; myrrh; pennyroyal;
peppermint; rosemary; sage; sarsaparilla; sassafras;
spearmint; tansy (?); valerian; wintergreen (?); wood
betony.

* * *

CATHARTIC: Has powerful laxative qualities;

Herbs exhibiting this quality: Aloe vera; elder (bark
or berries in quantity); fennel; mandrake.

* * *

CEPHALIC: Used in diseases, disorders and ailments
of the head;

Herbs exhibiting this quality: Rosemary.

* * *

CHOLAGOGUE: Controls/increases a deficient flow
of bile;

Herbs exhibiting this quality: Mandrake.

DECONGESTANT: Clears nose, nasal passages;

Herbs exhibiting this quality: Comfrey; garlic; ginger; golden seal; horsetail; vervain.

* * *

DEMULCENT: Soothes and relieves inflammation (similar to mucilaginous);

Herbs exhibiting this quality: Chickweed; coltsfoot; comfrey; fenugreek; ginseng; licorice; marshmallow; mullein; sarsaparilla; slippery elm; yellow dock.

* * *

DEOBSTRUCTANT, DEOBSTRUENT: Removes/dissolves obstructions from the organs;

Herbs exhibiting this quality: Fenugreek; golden seal; hawthorn; mandrake; plantain; vervain; wood betony.

* * *

DEPILATORY: Removes (body) hair (upon application to affected skin areas);

Herbs exhibiting this quality: Burdock root.

* * *

DEPURATIVE: Purifies system by removing waste toxins from body; purifies the blood:

Herbs exhibiting this quality: Burdock; cayenne; clover; dandelion; echinacea; fenugreek; garlic (?); horsetail; sanicle; vervain; yellow dock.

* * *

DETERGENT: Cleanses boils, wounds, carbuncles, etc.;

Herbs exhibiting this quality: Golden seal; horsetail; yellow dock.

* * *

DIAPHORETIC: Opens pores; improves/increases perspiration;

Herbs exhibiting this quality: Angelica; anise; bayberry; burdock; catnip; cayenne; black cohosh; blue cohosh; coltsfoot; echinacea; elder; elecampane; fennel; garlic; ginger (when taken hot); ginseng; horehound; hyssop; linden; lobelia; mandrake; pennyroyal; rosemary; sage (taken hot); sassafras spearmint; tansy; vervain; yarrow.

* * *

DISCUTIENT: Dissolves tumors; "reverses" (rather than "ripens") tumors;

Herbs exhibiting this quality: Chickweed; elder; sanicle; yellow dock.

* * *

DIURETIC: Promotes flow of urine; helps reduce excess water (and weight) within the system;

Herbs exhibiting this quality: Alfalfa; angelica; burdock; black cohosh; blue cohosh; cubeb berries; dandelion; elder; elecampane; fennel; garlic; golden seal; gotu kola; hops; horehound; horsetail; juniper berries; lobelia; marshmallow; masterwort; milkweed; mullein; nettle; plantain; sage (taken cool); St. Johnswort; sarsaparilla; sassafras; scullcap; self-heal; slippery elm; spearmint; uva ursi; wintergreen; yarrow.

\* \* \*

DRASTIC: Strong pronounced action;

Herbs exhibiting this quality: Aloe vera.

\* \* \*

EMETIC: Causes vomiting and purging;

Herbs exhibiting this quality: Bayberry (large amounts); cayenne; (large amounts); elder (bark in quantity); false unicorn (large amounts); milkweed; vervain; wintergreen.

\* \* \*

EMMENAGOGUE: Promotes/induces menstruation, menstrual flow;

Herbs exhibiting this quality: Aloe vera; angelica; catnip; cohosh (black — esp. if menses delayed by cold, exposure); blue cohosh; elecampane; ginger; horsetail; masterwort; myrrh; pennyroyal; rosemary; tansy; vervain; wintergreen.

* * *

EMOLLIENT: Softens, soothes, relieves inflamed areas, joints, etc;

Herbs exhibiting this quality: Aloe vera; coltsfoot; elder; marshmallow; mullein; slippery elm.

* * *

EXANTHEMATOUS: Heals the skin; affects skin diseases/eruptions (usually applied externally) such as measles, rash, etc.;

Herbs exhibiting this quality: Chickweed; elder.

* * *

EXPECTORANT: Expels, "breaks up" phlegm and mucus from respiratory system;

Herbs exhibiting this quality: Angelica; black cohosh; coltsfoot; comfrey; cubeb berries; elecampane; garlic; ginger; horsehound; hyssop; licorice; linden; lobelia; myrrh; pennyroyal; sage; sanicle; slippery elm; vervain.

* * *

FARINACEOUS: Has a starchy or mealy quality;

Herbs exhibiting this quality: Fenugreek.

* * *

FEBRIFUGE: Reduces fevers;

Herbs exhibiting this quality: Angelica; burdock;
calamus; cayenne; coltsfoot (?); fenugreek; gotu kola;
hops; hyssop; licorice; lobelia; nettle; pennyroyal;
sassafras; self-heal; vervain; witch hazel; yarrow.

* * *

FLAVORER/FLAVORANT: Used with other, less palatable
herbs to improve the flavor;

Herbs exhibiting this quality: Anise; fennel;
licorice; sassafras.

* * *

HEPATIC: Affects the liver; increases bile, digestive
juices and subsequently improves bowel movement;

Herbs exhibiting this quality: Dandelion; horehound;
horsetail.

* * *

HYPNOTIC: Alters consciousness; may induce sleep (mild
or trance-like), relaxation;

Herbs exhibiting this quality: Hops.

* * *

LAXATIVE: Bowel cleanser; promotes bowel action;

Herbs exhibiting this quality: Chaparral; chickweed;
cubeb; damiana; golden seal; hawthorn; horehound (large
doses); hyssop; licorice; mandrake; milkweed;
raspberry.

* * *

LINAMENT: Reaches deep into muscles, joints, through skin;

Herbs exhibiting this quality: Cayenne; wintergreen.

* * *

MUCILAGINOUS: Anti-inflammatory; soothes inflamed areas;

Herbs exhibiting this quality: Cayenne; chickweed; comfrey; fenugreek; marshmallow; plantain (seeds); slippery elm.

* * *

NARCOTIC: Creates sleep, lethargy and stupor; in excess, may cause comatose condition;

Herbs exhibiting this quality: Gotu kola (large doses).

* * *

NERVINE: Soothes/calms/quiets nerves, nervous irritation;

Herbs exhibiting this quality: Catnip; black cohosh; damiana; hops; horsetail; linden; lobelia; rosemary; sage; St. Johnswort; scullcap; valerian; vervain; wood betony.

* * *

NUTRIENT: Provides vitamins, minerals and other nutritional requirements;

Herbs exhibiting this quality: Alfalfa; cayenne; chickweed; comfrey; dandelion (leaves); hawthorn (often made into jelly); raspberry (fruit); rose hips; slippery elm.

* * *

OPTHALMIC/OPTHALMICUM: Affects the eyes (usually used as eyewash);

Herbs exhibiting this quality: Golden seal; marshmallow; rose/rose hips (rose water); rosemary; sarsaparilla.

* * *

PARTURIENT: Promotes/induces labor at childbirth;

Herbs exhibiting this quality: Raspberry.

* * *

PECTORAL: Produces effects in the chest area; relieves chest ailments;

Herbs exhibiting this quality: Anise; chickweed; coltsfoot; comfrey; fennel; hops (?); horehound; horsetail; lobelia; marshmallow; mullein; myrrh; nettle; rose/rose hips.

* * *

PREVENTIVE: Helps prevent disease;

Herbs exhibiting this quality: Garlic; ginger;
ginseng.

* * *

PUNGENT: Spicy; opens respiratory passages;

Herbs exhibiting this quality: Cayenne; garlic;
ginger; self-heal.

* * *

PURGATIVE: Profound laxative (bowel-clearing) effect;

Herbs exhibiting this quality: Cubeb berries;
milkweed; raspberry.

* * *

REFRIGERANT: Cools system; relieves thirst; cools
inflamed areas;

Herbs exhibiting this quality: Catnip; chickweed;
fennel; plantain; rose/rose hips; self-heal (?).

* * *

RELAXANT: Relieves muscular stress and tension;
calms nervousness; relaxes muscles;

Herbs exhibiting this quality: Anise; catnip;
chamomile; black cohosh; lobelia (in large doses).

* * *

RESOLVENT: Dissolves/removes tumors;

Herbs exhibiting this quality: Chickweed; mandrake; St. Johnswort.

* * *

RESTORATIVE: Helps heal/improve/restore those persons long-suffering from debilitating illnesses;

Herbs exhibiting this quality: Garlic; ginger; ginseng.

* * *

RUBEFACIENT: Improves circulation; reddens the skin;

Herbs exhibiting this quality: Bayberry; cayenne; elder; garlic; hyssop; nettle; sage; valerian.

* * *

SEDATIVE: Calms emotional imbalances; eases nervousness;

Herbs exhibiting this quality: Catnip; chamomile; black cohosh; damiana; hops; lobelia; mandrake; mullein; pennyroyal; plantain (seeds); rose/rose hips; St. Johnswort; saw palmetto berries; valerian; witch hazel.

* * *

SIALAGOGUE: Increases salivation;

Herbs exhibiting this quality: Cayenne; false unicorn; ginger; mandrake.

* * *

STIMULANT: Has a rapid, "energizing" quality;
improves appetite, outlook on life;

Herbs exhibiting this quality: Angelica; anise;
bayberry; catnip; cayenne; chamomile; clover (mild);
cubeb berries (mild); damiana; dandelion; elecampane;
false unicorn; fennel; garlic; ginger; ginseng; gotu
kola; hawthorn; horehound; hyssop; linden; lobelia (in
small amounts); masterwort; myrrh; pennyroyal;
peppermint; raspberry; rosemary; sage; sarsaparilla;
sassafras; spearmint; tansy; valerian; wintergreen;
yarrow.

* * *

STOMACHIC: Promotes digestion; improves appetite;
aids stomach, digestive disorders;

Herbs exhibiting this quality: Alfalfa; aloe vera;
anise; calamus; cayenne; chamomile; cubeb berries;
damiana; dandelion; elecampane; fennel; garlic; ginger;
ginseng; golden seal; hawthorn; hops; horsetail;
juniper berries; licorice; linden; myrrh; peppermint;
raspberry; rosemary; sassafras; spearmint; wood betony.

* * *

STYPTIC: Stops bleeding (e.g., from cuts, wounds);

Herbs exhibiting this quality: Cayenne; comfrey;
nettle; plantain; sanicle; self-heal; wintergreen;
witch hazel.

* * *

SUDORIFIC: Promotes profuse perspiration;

Herbs exhibiting this quality: Cayenne; garlic;
hyssop; pennyroyal; peppermint; sage; sarsaparilla (hot
tea); vervain; yarrow (?).

* * *

TONIC: A general strengthener; helps weak system heal
and improve; has a slow "energizing" quality (often
used as a regular beverage);

Herbs exhibiting this quality: Alfalfa; angelica;
anise; bayberry; calamus; catnip; cayenne; chamomile;
cohosh (black — esp. for mucous membranes); coltsfoot;
damiana; dandelion; elecampane; fenugreek; garlic;
ginger; ginseng; golden seal; hawthorn (esp. for
heart); hops; horehound; hyssop; licorice; milkweed;
myrrh; nettle; raspberry; rosemary; sage; sarsaparilla;
scullcap; self-heal; tansy; uva ursi; valerian;
vervain; witch hazel; wood betony; yarrow; yellow dock.

* * *

VERMIFUGE: Kills (esp. external) parasites (should be
applied locally, externally, for that function);

Herbs exhibiting this quality: Mandrake; self-heal;
tansy; vervain; yellow dock.

* * *

VULNERARY: Helps wounds, injuries heal;

Herbs exhibiting this quality: Aloe vera; bayberry;
burdock; calamus; chamomile; chickweed; comfrey;
garlic; golden seal; mullein; myrrh; plantain; St.
Johnswort; sanicle; self-heal; vervain; yarrow.

# SECTION III — TRADITIONAL OR HISTORICAL MEDICINAL USES FOR HERBS

**ARTHRITIC SYMPTOMS (Gout; rheumatism, aching joints etc.):**

Useful herbs: Anise; burdock; cayenne; chamomile; black cohosh; blue cohosh; fennel; fenugreek; ginseng; gotu kola; hawthorn (lumbago); hyssop; marshmallow (?); mullein; myrrh; nettle; pennyroyal (esp. gout); peppermint (esp. rheumatism, externally); plantain; sarsaparilla; sassafras; scullcap; self-heal; wintergreen; wood betony.

**BLEEDING/HEMORRHAGE (INTERNAL):**

Useful herbs: Bayberry; cayenne (?); comfrey; horsetail; mullein (esp. in lungs); nettle (esp. genitourinary, reproductive systems); plantain (?); sanicle; self-heal; witch hazel; yarrow.

**BLOOD DISORDERS/"CLEANSING":**

Useful herbs: Bayberry; burdock; cayenne; clover; dandelion; echinacea; elder; fenugreek; garlic; ginger; ginseng; golden seal (?); horsetail; licorice; mandrake; plantain (?); raspberry (?); rose (?); rosemary (?); St. Johnswort; sanicle (?); sarsaparilla (?); sassafras; self-heal (?); vervain; wintergreen (?); wood betony (?); yellow dock.

## BONE DISORDERS:

Useful herbs: Comfrey.


## BOWEL DISORDERS:

Useful herbs: Alfalfa; aloe vera; anise; catnip (esp. for enemas); cayenne; chamomile; chickweed; blue cohosh — esp. for colic, but should not be fed to infants; comfrey; cubeb berries; damiana; dandelion; elder; fennel; fenugreek; garlic; ginger; ginseng; golden seal; gotu kola; licorice; mandrake; marshmallow; milkweed; mullein; peppermint; raspberry; rose; sage; St. Johnswort; sanicle; sassafras; slippery elm; spearmint; tansy; wintergreen; witch hazel; wood betony.


## BURNS:

Useful herbs (usually applied externally): Aloe vera; burdock; chickweed; comfrey; elder; licorice; plantain; tansy; yarrow.


## CIRCULATORY DISORDERS:

Useful herbs: Bayberry; cayenne; chickweed; black cohosh; dandelion; garlic; ginger; ginseng; hawthorn; hyssop (?); licorice; mandrake; marshmallow (?); myrrh (if high cholesterol); peppermint; plantain; raspberry (?); rosemary; St. Johnswort; sarsaparilla; sassafras; saw palmetto (?); self-heal; tansy (?); vervain; wintergreen; witch hazel; yarrow; yellow dock.

COLDS AND INFLUENZA:

Useful herbs: Angelica; anise; cayenne; chamomile; chickweed; coltsfoot; comfrey; elder; elecampane; garlic; ginger; ginseng; golden seal; horehound; hyssop; juniper berries; licorice; linden; lobelia; mandrake; marshmallow; masterwort; mullein; myrrh; nettle; peppermint; rose; rosemary; sanicle (?); sarsaparilla; saw palmetto berries; slippery elm; tansy; vervain; wood betony; yarrow.

CONSTIPATION:

Useful herbs: Aloe vera; burdock; catnip; cayenne; chamomile; chickweed; cubeb berries damiana; dandelion (tea and salad); elder; fenugreek (?); garlic; golden seal; gotu kola; hyssop; licorice; mandrake.

COUGH:

Useful herbs: Clover; black cohosh; blue cohosh; coltsfoot; comfrey; cubeb berries; elecampane; fennel; garlic; ginger; ginseng; horehound; hyssop; juniper berries; licorice; linden; lobelia; mandrake; marshmallow; masterwort (?); milkweed; mullein; myrrh; peppermint; rose; rosemary; sanicle (?); sarsaparilla (?); sassafras (?); saw palmetto berries; slippery elm; vervain (?).

DIARRHEA (including dysentery):

Useful herbs: Bayberry; blueberry (leaves); chamomile
(?); comfrey; elder; garlic; ginger; hawthorn;
marshmallow; mullein; nettle; peppermint; plantain;
raspberry (esp. in infants); rose; slippery elm;
spearmint; witch hazel; yarrow.


DIGESTIVE DISORDERS: Disorders (including stomach,
liver, spleen, pancreas, small intestine, etc.):

Useful herbs: Alfalfa; aloe vera; anise; bayberry;
burdock; calamus; catnip; cayenne; chamomile;
chickweed; clover; comfrey; cubeb berries; damiana;
dandelion; elder; elecampane; false unicorn; fennel;
fenugreek; garlic; ginger; ginseng; golden seal;
hawthorn; hops; juniper berries; licorice; linden;
lobelia; mandrake; marshmallow; masterwort; milkweed;
myrrh; pennyroyal peppermint; raspberry; rose;
rosemary; sage; sanicle; sarsaparilla; sassafras;
slippery elm; spearmint; tansy; valerian; vervain;
wintergreen; wood betony; yarrow.


EAR/HEARING DIFFICULTIES:

Useful herbs for external use especially (as
eardrops): Angelica;

Internal use especially: Chamomile; hops.

## EYE DISORDERS:

Useful herbs for external use especially (as drops, eye wash, etc. — but also used internally): Angelica; chamomile; chickweed; fennel; golden seal; horsetail; marshmallow; plantain; rosemary; sarsaparilla; tansy.


## FEVER:

Useful herbs: Angelica; burdock; calamus; cayenne; coltsfoot; elecampane; fenugreek; ginseng (esp. recurring fevers, such as malaria); golden seal (?); gotu kola; hyssop; licorice; lobelia; nettle; pennyroyal; peppermint; sage; sarsaparilla; sassafras; self-heal; tansy; vervain; witch hazel; yarrow.


## GALLSTONES:

Useful herbs: Chamomile; comfrey (?) dandelion; garlic; ginger (?); mandrake (?); milkweed; sage (?); self-heal; wood betony (?).


## GAS, FLATULENCE:

Useful herbs: Angelica; anise; calamus; cayenne; chamomile; comfrey (?); cubeb berries; dandelion; fennel; garlic; ginger; ginseng; hyssop; juniper berries; mandrake (?); masterwort; myrrh; pennyroyal; peppermint; rosemary; sage; sarsaparilla; sassafras; spearmint; wintergreen; wood betony; yarrow.

GENITOURINARY DISORDERS (including kidneys, ureter tubes, urinary bladder, sexual/reproductive organs, etc):

Useful herbs: Alfalfa; burdock; chamomile; black cohosh; blue cohosh; comfrey; cubeb berries; damiana; dandelion; echinacea; elder; elecampane; false unicorn (?); fenugreek; garlic; ginger; ginseng; golden seal (esp. prostate problems); gotu kola (?); horsetail; hyssop; juniper; mandrake; marshmallow; masterwort; milkweed; mullein; nettle; plantain; raspberry; rosemary; sage; St. Johnswort; sanicle; sarsaparilla; sassafras; saw palmetto berries; slippery elm; spearmint; tansy; uva ursi; valerian; vervain; wintergreen; witch hazel; yarrow.


HEADACHE:

Useful herbs: Ginger; ginseng; pennyroyal; rosemary; scullcap; wood betony.


HEMORRHOIDS:

Useful herbs (usually applied externally): Aloe vera; burdock; chamomile; chickweed; coltsfoot; comfrey; garlic; golden seal; myrrh; nettle; plantain; spearmint; uva ursi; witch hazel; yarrow.

HYPERTENSION (High blood pressure):

Useful herbs: Black cohosh; blue cohosh; dandelion (?); garlic; ginseng (? — in moderation); hawthorn (?); hyssop; licorice (?); masterwort (?); myrrh; St. Johnswort (?); tansy.

INJURIES, ETC.:

Useful herbs for external use especially (as salves, packs, poultices, etc.): Aloe vera; burdock; cayenne; chickweed; clover; comfrey; elder; garlic (do not place directly on skin); horsetail; hyssop; licorice (?); marshmallow (esp. sprains, strains); mullein; nettle; pennyroyal (esp. bruises); plantain; raspberry; sage; St. Johnswort; sanicle; valerian; wintergreen (esp. sprains, strains, etc.);

Useful herbs for internal use especially: Calamus; chickweed; comfrey; garlic; nettle; plantain; sage (?); sanicle; self-heal; vervain; witch hazel; yarrow.

INSOMNIA:

Useful herbs: Anise; catnip; chamomile; damiana; dandelion; hops; lobelia; peppermint; scullcap; saw palmetto berries; valerian.

MENSTRUAL, MENOPAUSAL DISORDERS:

Useful herbs: Aloe vera; bayberry (leucorrhea); chamomile; black cohosh (esp. for delayed menses due to cold, exposure); blue cohosh; comfrey; cubeb berries (?); damiana (?); elecampane (delayed menses); garlic; ginger; ginseng (?); horehound; horsetail; juniper berries (esp. delayed menses); licorice (?); linden; masterwort; milkweed (?); myrrh; pennyroyal; plantain (?); raspberry; rosemary; St. Johnswort; sanicle (?); scullcap; slippery elm; tansy; uva ursi; vervain; wintergreen; witch hazel; yarrow (esp. excess bleeding).

NASAL CONGESTION, CATARRH:

Useful herbs: Bayberry; cayenne; coltsfoot; comfrey;
garlic; ginger; golden seal; horsetail; licorice;
marshmallow; mullein; myrrh (?); peppermint; rose (?);
sarsaparilla; sassafras (?); self-heal (?); slippery
elm (?); vervain (?).


NAUSEA:

Useful herbs: Anise; fennel (?); garlic; ginger;
ginseng (esp. "morning sickness" in pregnancy); golden
seal (esp. "morning sickness"); hawthorn (root);
licorice (?); pennyroyal; peppermint; raspberry;
spearmint.


NERVOUS (NERVE SYSTEM) DISORDERS:

Useful herbs: Anise; catnip; chamomile; clover;
damiana; elder (esp. epilepsy); ginseng; gotu kola;
hops; horsetail; juniper berries; linden; lobelia;
rosemary; sage; St. Johnswort; scullcap; valerian;
vervain.


PAIN; PAINFUL AILMENTS:

Useful herbs: Anise (?); catnip; chamomile; comfrey
(esp. breast tenderness); hops; licorice; marshmallow;
mullein; nettle; sassafras; valerian; wood betony (esp.
facial pain).

RESPIRATORY DISORDERS (including lungs, nasal passages, bronchial tubes, etc.):

Useful herbs: Angelica; anise; bayberry; cayenne; chamomile; chickweed; clover; coltsfoot; comfrey; cubeb beries; elecampane; garlic; ginger; ginseng; golden seal; horehound; hyssop; juniper berries; licorice; linden; lobelia; marshmallow; masterwort; milkweed; mullein; myrrh; nettle (esp. asthma); pennyroyal; peppermint; rose; sanicle; sarsaparilla; sassafras; saw palmetto; self-heal; slippery elm; vervain.

SEXUAL DISORDERS:

Useful herbs: Burdock; chamomile (eases sexual desire); black cohosh; blue cohosh; comfrey; cubeb berries; damiana (esp. low sex drive); echinacea; elder; false unicorn (?); garlic; ginger; ginseng (esp. for males); golden seal; gotu kola; hawthorn (swelling of genitals); juniper berries; mandrake; marshmallow; nettle; pennyroyal (esp. females); plantain; rosemary; sage (sexual balancer); St. Johnswort; sanicle (?); sarsaparilla (esp. venereal diseases) saw palmetto berries; tansy; uva ursi; vervain (?) wintergreen; witch hazel; yarrow.

## SKIN DISORDERS:

Useful herbs for external use (especially as salve, poultice, etc.): Aloe vera; chickweed; clover; coltsfoot; comfrey; elder; elecampane (esp. blemishes); fenugreek; garlic (do not place directly on skin); golden seal; hops; hyssop; plantain; St. Johnswort; sanicle; sassafras;

Useful herbs for internal use: Burdock; cayenne; comfrey (?); dandelion; garlic; golden seal; licorice (?); mullein; pennyroyal; plantain; sanicle; sarsaparilla; sassafras; self-heal; slippery elm; valerian; vervain; wintergreen; witch hazel (?); yarrow; yellow dock.

## STRESS AND TENSION; EMOTIONAL DISTRESS:

Useful herbs: Alfalfa; anise; catnip; chamomile; damiana; ginseng (?); hops; lobelia; mullein; pennyroyal; sage; St. Johnswort; scullcap (?).

## SWOLLEN GLANDS:

Useful herbs: Chamomile; dandelion; echinacea (?); ginseng (?); mullein; sarsaparilla; yellow dock.

THROAT, SORE THROAT:

Useful herbs (may be used internally or as poultices,
gargles, etc.): Bayberry (gargle); cayenne (poultice);
chickweed; coltsfoot; comfrey; echinacea; fenugreek;
golden seal; hops; horehound; hyssop; licorice; linden;
lobelia (?); mullein; myrrh; peppermint; raspberry;
rosemary; sage; sanicle; sarsaparilla (?); sassafras;
saw palmetto berries; self-heal; slippery elm.


TOOTH PROBLEMS:

Useful herbs: Alfalfa; bayberry (esp. gums); fennel
(esp. teething baby's gums); hops; mullein; myrrh;
rosemary; sanicle (?); sassafras; tansy.


TUMORS; ETC.:

Useful herbs (usually applied externally): Aloe vera
(?); chickweed (esp. poultice); coltsfoot (esp.
scrofulous tumors); comfrey (?); elder; hops; St.
Johnswort; sanicle; slippery elm; tansy; yellow dock.


WEAKNESS; "LOW ENERGY":

Useful herbs: Angelica; anise; bayberry; catnip;
cayenne; chamomile; damiana; dandelion; garlic; ginger;
ginseng; gotu kola; hyssop; licorice; rosemary (?);
sage; sarsaparilla (?); spearmint (?).

## WORMS, INTERNAL PARASITES:

Useful herbs: Aloe vera (?); catnip (?); cayenne (?); blue cohosh; false unicorn; garlic; horehound; hyssop; mandrake; nettle; sage; sarsaparilla; self-heal; tansy; vervain; wood betony.

# INDEX

Those words noted with an asterisk are herbal remedies.

# BIBLIOGRAPHY

The following publications have either been found to be useful for research or of reference value by the author and members of The G-Jo Institute.

Buchman, Dian Dincin. Dian Dincin Buchman's Herbal Medicine. New York: Gramercy Publishing Co., 1979.

Chinese Medicinal Herbs. San Francisco: Georgetown Press, 1973.

Culinary Herb & Spice Guide. Carolyn Heller West, Ed. Bronx, NY: VitaChart, 3130 Arlington Avenue, 1981.

Herbal Education Center. Herbs and Spices for Home Use (winter/spring 1981 catalog). Burlington, VT 05401: 6 Crescent Road.

Herbal Tea Guide. Carolyn Heller West, Ed. Bronx, NY: VitaChart, 1981.

Hyatt, Richard. Chinese Herbal Medicine. New York: Schocken Books, 1978.

Kloss, Jethro. Back to Eden. New York: Beneficial Books, 1972.

Meyer, Joseph E. The Herbalist. Clarence Meyer, Pub. No address, 1973.

Millspaugh, Chas. F.  American Medicinal Plants.  New
    York: Dover Pulications, Inc., 1974.

Thakkur, Dr. Chandrasekhar G. Herbal Cures. Bombay,
    India: Ancient Wisdom Publications, Sind Ayurvedic
    Pharmacy, 375 Kaleadevi Road, 1976.